Practical Medical English

实用医药英语

主 编 江晓东 谢家鑫 邬文婷

副主编 晏柳清 郑雪茜 陶 倩

编 者（以姓氏拼音为序）

陈琰晗 江晓东 吕 劼 庞 凌 冉凌云

陶 倩 王 化 王炎峰 伍满群 邬文婷

谢家鑫 晏柳清 殷汭君 余仕湖 郑雪茜

U0279966

重庆大学出版社

图书在版编目(CIP)数据

实用医药英语 / 江晓东等主编. –– 重庆:重庆大学
出版社,2018.12(2020.4重印)
高职高专商务英语系列教材
ISBN 978-7-5689-1097-2

Ⅰ.①实…　Ⅱ.①江…　Ⅲ.①医药学—英语—高等职
业教育—教材　Ⅳ.①R

中国版本图书馆 CIP 数据核字 (2018) 第 251167 号

实用医药英语

主编　江晓东　谢家鑫　邬文婷
责任编辑:张春花　　版式设计:牟　妮
责任校对:刘志刚　　责任印制:赵　晟

*

重庆大学出版社出版发行
出版人:饶帮华
社址:重庆市沙坪坝区大学城西路21号
邮编:401331
电话:(023) 88617190　88617185(中小学)
传真:(023) 88617186　88617166
网址:http://www.cqup.com.cn
邮箱:fxk@cqup.com.cn(营销中心)
全国新华书店经销
重庆共创印务有限公司印刷

*

开本:787mm×1092mm　1/16　印张:15.75　字数:380千
2019 年 1 月第 1 版　　2020 年 4 月第 3 次印刷
ISBN 978-7-5689-1097-2　定价:60.00元

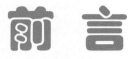

前 言
Preface

本书按照教育部高教司颁布的《高职高专教育英语教学基本要求》的相关内容，参考全国医护英语水平考试(METS)大纲的部分要求，针对职业院校医药专业学生的具体情况而编写。其目的是通过情景会话、专业阅读训练，培养学生在实际医药工作中综合应用英语的能力。

本书的编写针对医药类职业院校学生的英语基础学力和学习心理特点，以专门用途英语的相关理论为指导，把英语教学的新模式与医药科学的新知识、新进展、新观念有机整合；其内容新颖、充实，注重实用性和时代性，强化以学生发展为本的理念，适应课堂任务型教学，注重培养学生的自主学习能力。教材内容参照了职业教育与培训的新模式，力争与用人单位的实际需求接轨。

本书共10单元。对话部分以医护人员的实际工作经历为背景，先以医药相关图片引入，然后以医疗服务流程中常见情景为题材，句子实用易学，学习者可以根据这些对话，学会用英语准确流利地与患者沟通。课文主要以常见疾病为主题，介绍有关疾病的概念、症状、检查、治疗等。课后练习除了相关词汇练习及对课文的阅读理解练习之外，还有根据工作场景设计的相关会话、翻译、写作等任务型练习。全书附录有常见医学词汇的词干、前缀和后缀，医用缩略语和参考译文。

本书第一单元由王化（重庆三峡医药高等专科学校）编写；第二单元由晏柳清（重庆三峡医药高等专科学校）编写；第三单元由邬文婷（重庆三峡医药高等专科学校）编写；第四单元由吕劼（重庆医科大学附属第一医院）编写；第五单元由庞凌（重庆三峡医药高等专科学校）编写；第六单元由余仕湖（重庆三峡医药高等专科学校）编写；第七单元由郑雪茜（重庆三峡医药高等专科学校）编写；第八单元由陶倩（重庆三峡医药高等专科学校）编写；第九单元由伍满群（陆军军医大学附属第二医院）编写；第十单元由谢家

请登录重庆大学出版社网站（www.cqup.com.cn），搜索本书书名或书号，免费下载本书相关资源。

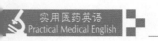
鑫（重庆三峡医药高等专科学校）编写；附录1由殷沩君（重庆三峡医药高等专科学校）编写；附录2由王炎峰（重庆医药高等专科学校）编写；附录3由陈琰晗（重庆医科大学护理学院）编写；附录4由冉凌云（昆明医科大学护理学院）；附录5、附录6和附录7由江晓东（重庆三峡医药高等专科学校）编写。

在本书的编写过程中，我们参阅了大量网上资料，并对这些资料的作者和提供者表示诚挚的谢意。同时，感谢编者所在单位和重庆大学出版社给予的大力支持和帮助。重庆三峡医药高等专科学校美籍志愿者Kreuzkamp Carolyn、澳大利亚籍英语教师Jason Shane Cahill和Cory James Peatey对每单元对话部分进行了审慎的校正，在此一并表示感谢。

由于时间紧迫和编者能力有限，书中可能还存在错漏之处，敬请使用者批评指正。

特别提示：本书所提供的信息不能替代专业医护咨询或诊治。缩略语仅供阅读英文专业材料时参考，非临床使用标准。

编　者

2018年10月

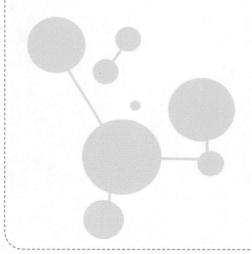

请登录重庆大学出版社网站（www.cqup.com.cn），搜索本书书名或书号，免费下载本书相关资源。

Contents

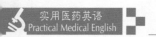

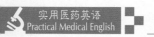

UNIT ONE

Learning Objectives

After studying this unit, you will be able to:

- ❑ Enlarge your vocabulary related to human organs;
- ❑ Talk about a medical college;
- ❑ Know how to receive a patient;
- ❑ Understand the relationship between chemistry and life;
- ❑ Understand the basic processes of life;
- ❑ Know some prefixes, suffixes or roots of medical terms about the orientational system;
- ❑ Write a school record and a table of pain rating and management.

Part 1   Pictures and Charts

Warming-up: Look at the following pictures, talk about them and then finish the task.

Picture 1

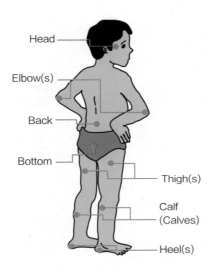

Head

Elbow(s)

Back

Bottom

Thigh(s)

Calf
(Calves)

Heel(s)

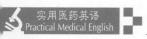

Picture 2

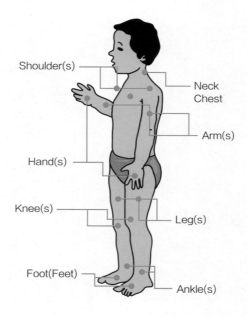

Picture 3

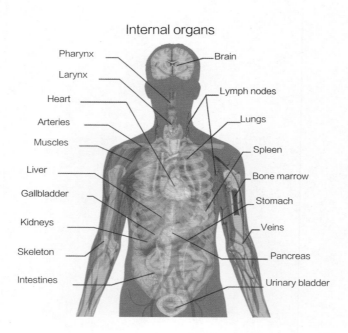

Task: Match the words in the left column with the explanations in the right column.

1. ankle	A. a muscular sac attached to the liver that stores bile (secreted by the liver) until it is needed for digestion
2. lymph node	B. the joint connecting the foot with the leg
3. gallbladder	C. a large gland behind the stomach which produces digestive enzymes and releases them into the duodenum
4. intestine	D. a small swelling in the lymphatic system where lymph is filtered and lymphocytes are formed
5. pancreas	E. the part of the alimentary canal between the stomach and the anus

Part 2 Listening and Speaking

Conversation A

Talking About Your College Life

(Li Mei, a student majoring in nursing, is introducing the medical college to her friend.)

Li Mei: Welcome to our college!

Wang Lan: What a beautiful campus! Is it newly built?

Li Mei: Yes. You can see the main teaching building, the labs, the imitation hospital and the library from here.

Wang Lan: How large the library is! How many teaching depart-ments are there in your college?

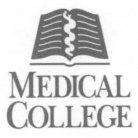

Li Mei: Five. They are the nursing department, the department of clinical medicine, the department of traditional Chinese medicine, the department of pharmaceutical sciences and the

pharmaceutical
/ˌfɑːməˈsjuːtɪkəl/
adj. 制药的

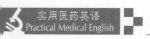
department which offers basic courses such as Chinese, English, and computer science.

Wang Lan: I see. What do the students learn in the nursing department?

Li Mei: The freshman students study subjects like biochemistry, anatomy and physiology. The sophomores study various nursing subjects, for example, fundamentals of nursing, medical nursing, surgical nursing…

Wang Lan: So is the study of these subjects enough for them to be a qualified nurse?

Li Mei: Absolutely not! Practice is also very important for them.

Wang Lan: Where do they practice?

Li Mei: The college provides many facilities for them to practice what they learn in the classroom. They can practice making beds, turning patients, performing sterilization procedures and other nursing skills in the imitation wards. What's more, before graduation, they have to work as student nurses in various departments of a general hospital.

Wang Lan: How long does it take them to do that?

Li Mei: At least ten months.

Wang Lan: That sounds interesting! They must be skillful nurses after they leave college.

Li Mei: Actually they have a long way to go before they become experienced nurses.

Wang Lan: Where can the students find jobs after they graduate?

Li Mei: Most of them will work in hospitals, first-aid centers, and other health care institutions.

Wang Lan: So you have a promising future! What you are going to do is valuable and meaningful.

Li Mei: Thank you! I hope so!

(335 words)

physiology /ˌfɪziˈɒlədʒɪ/ n. 生理学

sophomore /ˈsɒfəmɔː/ n. 大学二年级学生

fundamental /ˌfʌndəˈmentl/ n. 基本原则

surgical /ˈsɜːdʒɪkəl/ adj. 外科的

sterilization /sterɪlaɪˈzeɪʃən/ n. 杀菌

institution /ˌɪnstɪˈtjuːʃən/ n. 公共机构

Conversation B

Receiving a Patient

Task 1: Watch episode one and fill in the missing words referring to the original text. Then check your writing against the original one.

Doctor: Good morning. I am Doctor Stering. How can I help you?

Patient: Good morning, Doctor. I am Emily. I have had a ____ and ____ ____ since yesterday.

Doctor: Oh, did you take your temperature?

Patient: Yes, I did. The highest temperature was 39.8℃ at 11 p.m. last night. I took one pill of aspirin and felt much better.

Doctor: Any other symptoms?

Patient: I have a _____ _____ and_____, too.

Doctor: Ok, let me take your temperature first. Please keep this thermometer under your armpit for 5 minutes. Open your mouth and say "Ah", please. Your tonsils and larynx are red and swollen. Your temperature is 38.5° C. Your breathing sounds are normal and there is no problem with your lungs. You'd better take the_____ _____, Ok? This paper is for the lab test.

Patient: Sure. I really hope I can get better as soon as possible. See you later.

Task 2: Watch episode two and complete the answers according to the questions.

1. What does the result of blood test indicate?

The result indicates that the patient has an _____respiratory tract infection.

2. If fever persists, what should the patient do?

The patient should _____ if fever persists.

3. How many times should the patient take the medicine?

The patient should take it _____ a day.

Part 3   Reading Comprehension

Text A

Chemistry Is Life

Are you aware of the fact that every living thing is dependent

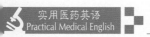
upon chemistry for life? This fact will be more clearly understood when you become aware that all the materials of plant and animal life and all the changes that occur in plants and animals are chemical in nature. In fact, chemistry is the science which deals with the composition of all materials and the changes which those materials undergo.

The human body is a chemical manufacturing plant. The food that is so essential to supplying energy and to building tissue in our bodies must be made soluble through the chemical processes of digestion. The food made soluble by digestion can supply energy and build tissue only through chemical processes which are carried on within the body cells. The glands of your body manufacture substances which are distributed to all parts of the body. These substances may determine such important characteristics as whether you are normal or subnormal in intelligence and whether you are fat or thin. Moreover, your nervous system, which makes it possible for you to distinguish between hot and cold, provides you with a sense of smell and makes it possible for you to use, feel and think, is dependent upon chemical reactions.

tissue /ˈtɪʃuː/ *n.* 组织

soluble /ˈsɒljʊbl/ *adj.* 可溶的

gland /glænd/ *n.* 腺体

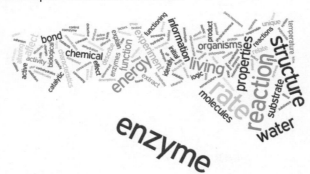

The close relationship between chemistry and plant life may easily be shown. Plants could not exist unless certain chemical changes occurred. Chemical changes within the plant make possible the absorption of carbon dioxide from the air and the use of it in the manufacture of food and of other plant cells. As this process is being carried on, oxygen, which is essential to all animal life, is related to the air. Through these chemical changes, man and all animal life are assured food and oxygen. Thus, plants make life possible.

dioxide /daɪˈɒksaɪd/ *n.* 二氧化物

All common products used every day for the preservation and protection of life are chemical products. The drugs which doctors prescribe for curing diseases, the antiseptics you use to prevent or hinder infection, the toothpaste you use to keep your teeth clean, the soap which assures body cleanliness, are the products of chemical laboratories.

prescribe /prɪsˈkraɪb/ *vt.* 给······开药
antiseptic /ˌæntɪˈseptɪk/ *n.* 消毒剂
hinder /ˈhɪndə/ *v.* 防止

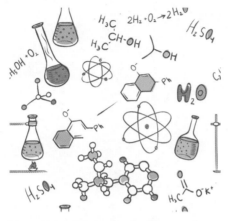

Industries, through the knowledge and use of chemistry, have provided many products which make life more pleasant and convenient. Among these products are nylon, metallic alloys and plastics, to name but a few.

(385 words)

nylon /ˈnaɪlɒn/ *n.* 尼龙
metallic /mɪˈtælɪk/ *adj.* 金属的
alloy /ˈælɔɪ/ *n.* 合金

Text B

Body Structure and Function

Anatomy deals with the structure and function of the human body. The study of anatomy makes you understand the basic concepts and principles of each organ system and how it contributes to maintaining homeostasis in the body.

Human beings are the most complicated organisms in this world. Imagine billions of microscopic parts, each with its own identity, working together in an organized manner for the existence of the total being. The human body is made up of billions of smaller structures of four major kinds.

Cells are defined as the simplest units of living matter that can

anatomy /əˈnætəmi/ *n.* 解剖学
homeostasis /ˌhəumɪəˈsteɪsɪs/ *n.* 动态平衡
complicated /ˈkɒmplɪkeɪtɪd/ *adj.* 复杂的
microscopic /ˌmaɪkrəˈskɒpɪk/ *adj.* 精微的
identity /aɪˈdentɪti/ *n.* 特性

maintain life and reproduce themselves. The human body, which consists of numerous cells, begins as a single, newly fertilized cell. Various cells exist in the human body, such as white blood cell, red blood cell, and platelet.

fertilize /'fɜːtɪlaɪz/
vt. 使受精

Tissues are somewhat more complex units than cells. By definition, a tissue is an organization of a great many similar cells with varying amounts and kinds of nonliving, intercellular substance among them.

definition /ˌdefɪ'nɪʃən/
n. 定义
intercellular /ˌɪntə'seljʊlə/
adj. 细胞间的

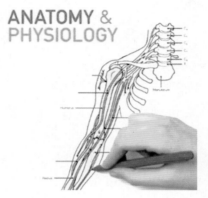

ANATOMY &
PHYSIOLOGY

epithelial /ˌepɪ'θiːlɪəl/
adj. 上皮的
lining /'laɪnɪŋ/ n. 内层
skeletal /'skelɪtl/
adj. 骨骼的
muscular /'mʌskjʊlə/
adj. 肌肉的
endocrine /'endəʊkrɪn/
n. 内分泌
cardiovascular
/ˌkɑːdɪəʊ'væskjʊlə/
adj. 心脏血管的
lymphatic /lɪm'fætɪk/
adj. 淋巴的
respiratory /rɪ'spɪrətəri/
adj. 呼吸的
digestive /daɪ'dʒestɪv/
adj. 消化的
urinary /'jʊərɪnəri/
adj. 泌尿的
reproductive
/ˌriːprə'dʌktɪv/
adj. 生殖的
physiological
/ˌfɪzɪə'lɒdʒɪkəl/
adj. 生理学的
psychological
/ˌsaɪkə'lɒdʒɪkəl/
adj. 心理学的
survival /sə'vaɪvəl/
n. 生存
constancy /'kɒnstənsi/
n. 恒久不变的状态

An organ refers to an organization of several different kinds of tissues so arranged that together they can perform a special function. For example, the stomach is an organization of muscle, connective, epithelial, and nervous tissues. Muscle and connective tissues form its wall; epithelial and connective tissues form its lining; and nervous tissue extends throughout both its wall and its lining.

Systems are the most complex of the component units of the human body. A system is an organization of varying numbers and kinds of organs so arranged that together they can perform complex functions for the body. Ten major systems compose the human body, namely, skeletal, muscular, nervous, endocrine, cardiovascular, lymphatic, respiratory, digestive, urinary and reproductive.

Body functions are the physiological or psychological functions of body systems. Survival is the body's most important business. Survival depends on the body's maintaining or restoring homeostasis, a state of relative constancy, of its internal environment.

Homeostasis depends on the body's ceaselessly carrying on

many activities. Its major activities or functions are responding to changes in the body's environment, exchanging materials between the environment and cells, metabolizing foods, and integrating all of the body's diverse activities.

metabolize /mə'tæbəlaɪz/
v. 使新陈代谢

The body's ability to perform many of its functions changes gradually over the years. In general, the body performs its functions least well at both ends of life—in infancy and old age. During childhood, body functions gradually become more and more efficient and effective. During late maturity and old age the opposite is true. During young adulthood, they normally operate with maximum efficiency and effectiveness.

infancy /'ɪnfənsi/
n. 幼年

maturity /mə'tʃʊərɪti/
n. 成熟
adulthood /'ædʌlthʊd/
n. 成人期

(429 words)

Text C

Life Process

The basic processes of life include organization, metabolism, responsiveness, movements, and reproduction. In humans, there are additional requirements such as growth, differentiation, respiration, digestion, and excretion. All of these processes are interrelated and function together to maintain individual life. Disease and death represent a disruption of the balance in these processes. The following is a brief description of the life process.

metabolism
/mə'tæbəlɪzəm/
n. 新陈代谢
differentiation
/ˌdɪfəˌrenʃɪ'eɪʃ ən/
n. 分化
respiration /ˌrespə'reɪʃ ən/
n. 呼吸
digestion /daɪ'dʒestʃ ən/
n. 消化
interrelated /ɪntərɪ'leɪtɪd/
adj. 相关的
disruption /dɪs'rʌpʃ ən/
n. 破坏

Organization

At all levels of the organizational scheme, there is a division of labor. Each component has its own job to perform in cooperation with others. Even a single cell, if it loses its integrity or organization, will die.

component /kəm'pəʊnənt/
n. 成分
integrity /ɪn'tegrɪti/
n. 完整

Metabolism

Metabolism includes all the chemical reactions that occur in the body. One phase of metabolism is catabolism in which complex substances are broken down into simpler building blocks and energy is released.

catabolism /kə'tæbəlɪzəm/
n. 分解代谢

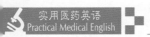
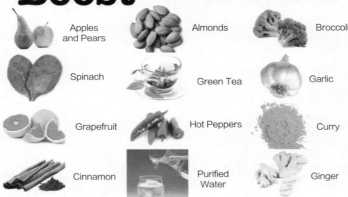

Boost Your Metabolism

Apples and Pears　Almonds　Broccoli

Spinach　Green Tea　Garlic

Grapefruit　Hot Peppers　Curry

Cinnamon　Purified Water　Ginger

Responsiveness

Responsiveness or irritability is concerned with detecting changes in the internal or external environments and reacting to that change. It is the act of sensing a stimulus and responding to it.

irritability /ˌɪrɪtəˈbɪlətɪ/ n. 过敏
stimulus /ˈstɪmjʊləs/ n. 刺激
cellular /ˈseljʊlə/ adj. 细胞的
molecule /ˈmɒlɪkjuːl/ n. 分子
diaphragm /ˈdaɪəfræm/ n. 横膈膜

Movement

There are many types of movement within the body. On the cellular level, molecules move from one place to another. Blood moves from one part of the body to another. The diaphragm moves with every breath.

Reproduction

Life is transmitted from one generation to the next through the reproduction of the organism. In a broader sense, reproduction also refers to the formation of new cells for the replacement and repair of old cells as well as for growth.

replacement /rɪˈpleɪsmənt/ n. 代替

Growth

Growth refers to an increase in size either through an increase in the number of cells or through an increase in the size of each cell. For growth to occur, anabolic processes must occur at a faster rate than catabolic processes.

anabolic /əˈnæbəlɪk/ adj. 合成代谢的

Differentiation

Differentiation is a developmental process by which unspecialized cells change into specialized cells with distinctive structural and functional characteristics. Through differentiation,

distinctive /dɪsˈtɪŋktɪv/ adj. 有特色的

cells develop into tissues and organs.

Respiration

Respiration refers to all the processes involved in the exchange of oxygen and carbon dioxide between the cells and the external environment.

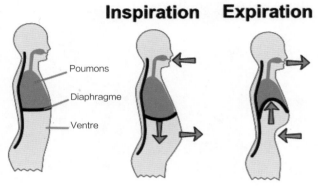

Digestion

Digestion is the process of breaking down complex ingested foods into simple molecules that can be absorbed into the blood and utilized by the body.

Excretion

Excretion is the process that removes the waste products of digestion and metabolism from the body. It gets rid of by-products that the body is unable to use, many of which are toxic and incompatible with life.

In addition to the processes described above, life depends on certain physical factors from the environment. These include water, oxygen, nutrients, heat, and pressure.

(427 words)

excretion /ɪkˈskriːʃən/
n. 排泄

toxic /ˈtɒksɪk/
adj. 有毒的
incompatible
/ˌɪnkəmˈpætəbl/
adj. 不调和的
nutrient /ˈnjuːtriənt/
n. 营养物

Exercises

Task 1　Oral Practice

Direction: Introduce one medical subject you have studied or are studying to your partner.
　　　　　You can use the following information as reference.

Course Name: Physiology　　　*Theory Hours:* 26　　　*Lab Hours:* 10

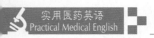

Description:

1. According to the Chinese educational guideline, this course studies the basic principles of human physiology.

2. The subject includes the presentation on the anatomical organization and the physiological functions of central and peripheral nervous systems, skeletal and smooth muscle, cardiovascular, respiratory, renal systems, endocrine and reproductive systems.

3. The course is taken before clinical courses.

Major Topics:

Foundation of Cells; Blood; Blood Circulation; Respiration; Digestion and Absorption; Energy Metabolism and Temperature; Elimination; Endocrine System and Reproductive System; Neurological System; Sensory System…

Task 2   Vocabulary Exercise

Direction: Fill in the blanks with the following words. Change the forms if necessary.

excrete	component	toxic	malnutrition	fertilize
cellular	respiration	digest	irritable	mature

1. Food is _____ in the stomach and bowels so that it can be used in the body.

2. Waste matter and sweat are _____ from the human body.

3. The insecticide should be kept beyond children's reach because it is_____.

4. Many children in Africa are suffering from starvation because of _____.

5. A _____ phone is also called a mobile phone, or a handphone.

6. His body and character _____ during these years.

7. They failed to find the _____ egg in the patient's body.

8. Artificial _____ is very crucial in first-aid.

9. Each _____ of human body has its own job to perform.

10. Some patients with mental illness tend to be _____.

Task 3   Reading Comprehension

Direction: Choose the best answer to finish each statement according to Text A and Text B.

1. _____ do not belong to the four basic human body structure units.

   A. Cells   B. Differentiations   C. Tissues   D. Systems

2. The name _____ is suggested for the relatively constant states maintained by the body.

   A. homoeosis   B. homogenization   C. homology   D. homeostasis

3. One of the additional requirements specific to the basic processes of human life is _____.

   A. organization   B. differentiation   C. metabolism   D. responsiveness

4. One phase of metabolism is _____ in which complex substances are broken down into simpler building blocks and energy is released.

   A. organization   B. responsiveness   C. catabolism   D. growth

5. Responsiveness or _____ is concerned with detecting changes in the internal or external environments and reacting to that change.

   A. flexibility   B. contractility   C. irritability   D. responsibility

Task 4   Translation

Direction: Put the following passage into Chinese with the help of your dictionary.

This course is an introduction to the structure and function of the human body. It provides students with a solid foundation in human anatomy and physiology, including many of the real-world associated diseases, conditions and applications, and an emphasis on how various organ systems maintain homeostasis. It incorporates various activities and experiments. The use of core and advanced biology equipment is required such as microscopes, human models, and prepared slides of the various body sectors. The college offers an excellent internet site with interactive activity links, student quizzes, and teacher resources.

Task 5   Prefixes, Suffixes and Roots

Direction: Learn the prefixes, suffixes or roots in the table and then choose the best answers.

Orientational System (方位系统)

汉语 / 英语	常用词根	例词
上 up	epi- super- supra-	epicytoma 上皮瘤；epiderm 表皮；epinephrine 肾上腺素 superconductor 超导体 supraaortic 上主动脉；supraclavicular 锁骨上的； supracapsulin 肾上腺素

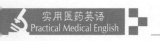
(Continued)

汉语 / 英语	常用词根	例词
下 down	infer(o)- infra- sub- hypo-	inferolateral 下外侧的 infraorbital 眶下的；infraauricular 耳下的 subaxillary 腋下的；subcutaneous 皮下的 hypodermic 皮下的
左 left	leva- levo-	levamizole 左旋咪唑 levocardiogram 左侧心电图
右 right	dextr(o)-	dextrocardiogram 右侧心电图；dextrocular 惯用右眼的 dextrocardia (dexiocardia) 右位心
前 front	ante- pre- pro	antenatal 产前的 preoperative 术前的；precordium 心前区 prostatic 前列腺的；prophylaxis 预防法
后 behind	post retr(o)-	postpartum 产后的；post-operative 术后的 retrobulbar 眼球后的；retrobronchial 支气管后的
内 inside	endo- intra-	endocardium 心内膜；endocrine 内分泌的 intravenous 静脉内的；intramuscular 肌肉内的； intrauterine 子宫内
外 outside	ect(o)- exo- extra	ectohormone 外激素 exocervix 外子宫颈 extraarticular 关节外的；extracorporeal 体外的； extracranial 颅外的
中心 center	centro-	centrocyte 中央细胞；centrokinesis 中枢性运动
中间 middle	medi(o)-	media 介质，血管中层；mediocidin 中霉素
周围 around	circum-; peri-	circumcision 包皮环切术；periodontitis 牙周炎

1. The word meaning "of the area beneath the skin" is _____.

   A. hypotension   B. hypodermic   C. hypothermia   D. hypothyriod

2. On or of the outside is called _____.

   A. extent   B. extant   C. extinct   D. external

3. The Chinese equivalent to the word "endocardium" is _____.

   A. 心内膜   B. 内分泌   C. 子宫颈内   D. 囊内的

4. The correct spelling for the word " 中枢性运动 " is _____.

    A. centriole   B. centrocyte   C. centrokinesis   D. centroplasm

5. The English term for " 眼球后的 " is _____.

    A. retrocecal   B. retrobulbar   C. retrocavalureter   D. retrocolic

6. What is the Chinese term for "levocardiogram"?

    A. 左旋甲状腺素   B. 左位心   C. 左旋咪唑   D. 左侧心电图

7. The English term for " 肘前的 " is _____.

    A. antecubital   B. antebrachial   C. antecubital   D. anteflexion

8. The Chinese term for "circumanal" is _____.

    A. 阑尾周围的   B. 包皮环切术   C. 肛门周围的   D. 眼周围的

9. The Chinese term for "dextrocular" is _____.

    A. 右位心   B. 惯用右眼的   C. 右心电图   D. 右旋

10. What is the Chinese term for "supracapsulin"?

    A. 锁骨上   B. 主动脉上的   C. 视交叉上的   D. 肾上腺素

Task 6   Practical Writing

Direction: Read the following practical writing samples carefully and then design a similar school record or a table of pain rating and management by yourself.

Sample 1

School Record

Name: Lin Ran   Gender: Female   Date of Birth: 05/07/1988 Major: Nursing

Grade: 2005 Class: 1 Date of Entrance: 09/01/2005 Date of Graduation: 07/10/2008

Semester	Course	Score	Semester	Course	Score
The First Semester	Chemistry	92	The Third Semester	Medical Nursing	84
	Biology	90		Surgical Nursing	89
	Anatomy	88		Nursing Fundamentals	84
	Physiology	90		Nursing Skills	80
	Aesthetics	85		Community Nursing	73
	Politics	85		Medical Psychology	76
	English	88		English	80
	PE	80		PE	88

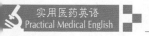

(Continued)

Semester	Course	Score	Semester	Course	Score
The Second Semester	Biochemistry	80	The Fourth Semester	Gyn. and Ob. Nursing	86
	Microbiology	73		E.E.N.T Nursing	84
	Pathology	76		Pediatric Nursing	84
	Pharmacology	80		Geriatric Nursing	89
	Politics	88		Psychiatric Nursing	84
	English	86		Lemology	90
	PE	84		PE	90

Practical Courses:

Semester	Course	Period	Evaluation
The Fifth Semester to the Sixth Semester	Medical Nursing	8 weeks	Pass
	Psychiatric Nursing	3 weeks	Pass
	Pediatrics Nursing	3 weeks	Pass
	Operation Room	4 weeks	Pass
	Surgical Nursing	8 weeks	Pass
	Gyn.& Ob. Nursing	4 weeks	Pass
	Emergency Nursing	3 weeks	Pass
	ICU Nursing	3 weeks	Pass

Sample 2

Pain Rating and Management

0	1	2	3	4	5	6	7	8	9	10
No pain										Worst pain imaginable

Date	Time	Pain rating (0–10)	Pain medication (name, dose, how often taken)	Other pain–relief methods tried	Side effects from pain medication
6/8 (example)	8 a.m.	8	Morphine 30 mg every 4 hrs	massage	constipation

UNIT TWO

Learning Objectives

After studying this unit, you will be able to:

- ❏ Enlarge your vocabulary related to hospital departments;
- ❏ Talk about a hospital;
- ❏ Know how to consult a doctor;
- ❏ Know something about diet;
- ❏ Know something about common respiratory diseases such as cold and pneumonia;
- ❏ Know some prefixes, suffixes or roots of medical terms about the respiratory system;
- ❏ Write an application letter and a medication template.

Part 1   Pictures and Charts

Warming-up: Look at the following pictures, talk about them and then finish the task.

Picture 1

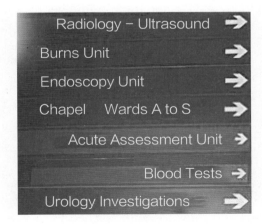

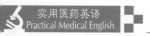
Picture 2

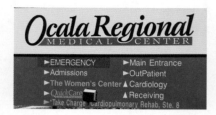

Picture 3

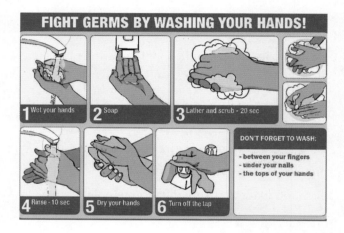

Task: Arrange the following sentences in the correct order according to Picture 3.

A. Dry your hands with a clean towel. Get a clean, dry towel to dry your hands or use an air drying unit to dry them. Dry your hands completely.

B. Wet your hands with water. Allow your hands to get wet all over.

C. Rinse your hands thoroughly. After you finish lathering and scrubbing your hands, place your hands under the running water again and allow the water to run over them. Rinse away all of the soap from your hands.

D. Apply enough soap to cover all hand surfaces. You can use a bottle of liquid hand soap, a soap bar, or powdered soap.

E. Keep washing your hands for 20 seconds or more. Rub hands palm to palm: right palm over left thumb dorsum with interlaced fingers and vice versa; palm to palm with fingers interlaced; backs of fingers to opposing palms with fingers interlocked; rotational rubbing of left thumb clasped in right palm and vice versa; rotational rubbing, backwards and forwards with clasped fingers of right hand in left palm and vice versa.

F. Use a towel to turn off the faucet. You can also use your elbow to turn off the faucet if a towel is not available.

Part 2   Listening and Speaking

Conversation A

Introducing the Hospital

(Meimei, a nurse, is introducing the hospital where she is working to her friend Lily.)

Meimei: Good news! I've found a job in Xinhua Hospital!

Lily: Congratulations! What kind of hospital is it?

Meimei: A general hospital. It's also a teaching hospital because it's attached to a medical college.

Lily: Where is the hospital?

Meimei: The hospital is located downtown. It's very convenient to get there.

Lily: Is it a large hospital?

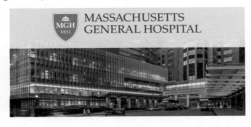

Find a Doctor

Appointments & Referrals

Patient & Visitor Info

Patient Gateway

Contact Us

Maps & Directions

Meimei: Yes. There are 1,200 beds and 500 medical workers.

Lily: What kind of doctors and nurses do you have?

Meimei: We have many kinds of doctors, such as physicians, surgeons, dentists, ENT (ear, nose and throat) doctors. There are

physician /fɪˈzɪʃ ən/
n. 内科医生
surgeon /ˈsɜːdʒən/
n. 外科医生
dentist /ˈdentɪst/
n. 牙科医生

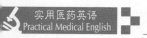

also many head nurses, nurses and midwives.

Lily: How many offices and departments are there in the hospital?

Meimei: A great deal! In the outpatient department, there are registration offices, pharmacy, consulting rooms, injection rooms and daytime wards.

Lily: And you also have an inpatient department?

Meimei: Sure! In the inpatient department, we have an internal medicine department, surgical department, ICU (intensive care unit), operating theatre and some other departments. In each department, there are many wards.

Lily: What do you specifically do for your patients?

Meimei: I take their temperatures and pulses, give them injections, fluid transfusions and blood transfusions. I make their beds. I give them medicine as doctors prescribe. I…

Lily: I see. It must be a very interesting and important job.

Meimei: Sure, it is. However, it's also very tiring. Any minor mistake in clinical work will not be tolerated. Also, the weekly night shift really disturbs my sleep habits.

Lily: I understand. Care for yourself first, so that you can care for your patients! I hope you will get used to your job as soon as possible. See you!

Meimei: Thank you! It's been nice talking with you. See you!

(306 words)

midwife /ˈmɪdwaɪf/
n. 助产士

pharmacy /ˈfɑːməsi/
n. 药房

injection /ɪnˈdʒekʃən/
n. 注射
transfusion /trænsˈfjuːʒən/
n. 输液

Conversation B

Consulting a Doctor

Task 1: Watch episode one and fill in the missing words referring to the original text. Then check your writing against the original.

Doctor: Hi, I am Doctor Susan. How can I help you?

Patient: Hi, doctor. I am Mary. Would you please take a look at my lab result?

Doctor: Sure. Take a seat, please.

Patient: Thank you. This is the blood result of my _____ _____ , and the other is the _____ _____ .

Doctor: I see. I'd like to know your medical history first. Have you had any problems with your kidney or liver?

Patient: Yes. I was told I had IgA nephropathy five years ago because both my uric acid and creatinine were too high. My urine has been tea-colored for almost five years.

Doctor: Did you have a _____?

Patient: No. The doctor suggested the biopsy but I am really afraid of that. So they haven't been able to diagnose the IgA until now.

Doctor: What kind of symptoms do you have now?

Patient: Oh, I have had gout for a week, and my left foot is still _____ and _____.

Task 2: Watch episode two and complete the answers according to the questions.

1. What is the patient taking for gout these days?

The patient is taking a _____.

2. Why the patient should avoid the painkillers?

Because the pain killers affect _____.

3. What's the doctor's suggestion?

The doctor suggests trying some _____.

Part 3   Reading Comprehension

Text A

You Are What You Eat

Our bodies are very complex. We can maintain ourselves and perform our normal functions only within a limited temperature range. As you know, the normal temperature of an adult human being is 37 ℃. This temperature must be maintained by the body in spite of external temperature changes. To do this, the body must produce heat and enough energy to enable it to perform important biological processes, such as muscular motion, digestion, breathing, circulation of blood, etc. To obtain this energy, everyone eats or takes in food. After hundreds of complex chemical processes, the foods we eat become the substances necessary for the normal functioning of the human body. Foods are also required in building

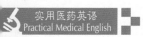

new tissue and in repairing broken-down or worn-out cells.

In the course of your lifetime, you will probably consume some fifty tons of food or so. The chief nutrients found in them are carbohydrates, fats and oils, proteins, minerals, and vitamins. Water, even though it does not produce energy, is absolutely essential for the proper working of your body. Any lack of it will upset the proper concentrations of the various fluids in your body and will cause many organs to fail to function normally.

carbohydrate
/ˌkɑːbəʊˈhaɪdreɪt/
n. 碳水化合物
protein /ˈprəutiːn/
n. 蛋白质
fluid /fluːɪd/ n. 流体

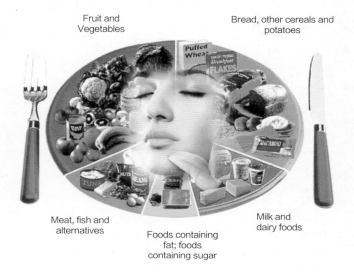

Fruit and Vegetables

Bread, other cereals and potatoes

Meat, fish and alternatives

Foods containing fat; foods containing sugar

Milk and dairy foods

Carbohydrates make up part of our diet. A carbohydrate is an organic compound composed of carbon, hydrogen and oxygen. In a carbohydrate, hydrogen and oxygen are present in the same proportion as in water, that is, two atoms of hydrogen to one of oxygen. The most common carbohydrates are the sugars and the starches.

Fats and oils are also component parts of our diet. These nutrients contain carbon, hydrogen and oxygen in varying proportions. Animal and vegetable fats and oils are mixtures of esters, which are liquid under normal conditions and are called oils; those which are solid are generally called fats. They serve as secondary sources of energy in the body, and also as breaking parts for various tissues.

organic /ɔːˈgænik/
adj. 有机的
carbon /ˈkɑːbən/
n. 碳
hydrogen /ˈhaɪdrədʒən/
n. 氢
oxygen /ˈɒksɪdʒən/
n. 氧
atom /ˈætəm/ n. 原子
starch /stɑːtʃ/ n. 淀粉
ester /ˈestə/ n. 酯

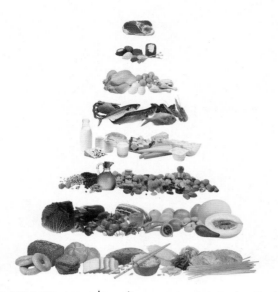

Proteins are very complex nitrogen compounds. Carbohydrates and fats are the chief sources of energy used in the activities of the body, but they are not the chief substances of which active body tissues are composed. Muscle tissue, for example, contains but little carbohydrate and often very little fat. The chief elements of the muscles and the protoplasm of plant and animal cells generally are compounds called proteins. Proteins are distinguished from carbohydrates and fats by the presence of nitrogen, for proteins contain about 16% of nitrogen.

The minerals of the body build up more than 4% of the weight of the body. Animal tissues contain compounds of many kinds of inorganic substances, which are obtained from foods. These foods become part of different body tissues.

Vitamins are substances that your body needs to grow and develop normally. Each vitamin has specific jobs. If you have low levels of certain vitamins, you may get health problems. For example, if you don't get enough vitamin C, you could become anemic. The best way to get enough vitamins is to eat a balanced diet with a variety of foods. In some cases, you may need to take vitamin supplements. It's a good idea to ask your health care provider first. High doses of some vitamins can cause problems.

(542 words)

nitrogen /ˈnaɪtrədʒən/ n. 氮

protoplasm /ˈprəʊtəplæzəm/ n. 原生质

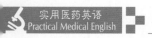
Text B

Common Cold

The common cold, also known as an upper respiratory tract infection, is a contagious illness that can be caused by a number of different types of viruses. Because of the great number of viruses that can cause a cold and because new cold viruses develop, the body never builds up resistance against all of them. For this reason, colds are a frequent and recurring problem.

tract /trækt/ n.（连通身体组织或器官的）道
infection /ɪnˈfekʃən/ n. 感染
contagious /kənˈteɪdʒəs/ adj. 传染性的
virus /ˈvaɪərəs/ n. 病毒
recur /rɪˈkɜː/ vi. 复发

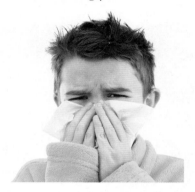

Symptoms of a common cold include nasal stuffiness and drainage, sore throat, hoarseness, cough, and perhaps a fever and headache. Many people with a cold feel tired and achy. These symptoms typically last for 3 to 10 days.

drainage /ˈdreinidʒ/ n. 引流
typically /ˈtɪpɪkli/ adv. 通常

Colds often get better within a few days to weeks, whether you take medication or not. However, a cold virus can pave the way for other infections to invade the body, including sinus or ear infections, and bronchitis. If you have asthma, chronic bronchitis, or emphysema, your symptoms may be worsened for many weeks even after your cold has gone away.

sinus /ˈsaɪnəs/ n. 窦
bronchitis /brɒŋˈkaɪtɪs/ n. 支气管炎
asthma /ˈæsmə/ n. 哮喘
chronic /ˈkrɒnɪk/ adj. 慢性的
emphysema /ˌemfɪˈsiːmə/ n. 肺气肿

The common cold is spread mostly by hand-to-hand contact. For example, a person with a cold blows or touches his or her nose and then touches someone else who then becomes infected with the virus. Additionally, the cold virus can live on objects such as pens, books, and coffee cups and can be acquired from such objects. While common sense would suggest that coughing and sneezing spread the common cold, these are actually very poor mechanisms for spreading a cold.

mechanism /ˈmekənɪzəm/ n. 机制

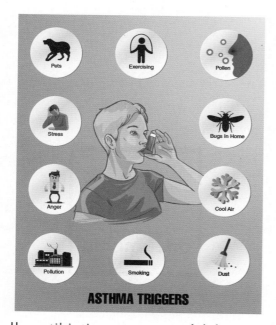

ASTHMA TRIGGERS

Generally antibiotics are not useful for treating a cold. Antibiotics only work against illnesses caused by bacteria and colds are often caused by viruses. Not only do antibiotics not help, but they can also cause allergic reactions that may be fatal. Further, using antibiotics when they are not necessary has led to the growth of several strains of common bacteria that have become resistant to antibiotics. For these and other reasons, it is important to limit the use of antibiotics to situations in which they are necessary. Sometimes, an infection with bacteria can follow the cold virus. Bacterial complications that arise from common cold are treated with antibiotics.

Several treatments can ease the symptoms associated with a common cold. Decongestants and nasal sprays can help reduce symptoms. People with heart disease, poorly controlled high blood pressure, or other illness should contact their physician prior to using these medications. Additionally, over-the-counter nasal sprays should not be used for more than three days because the nose can become dependent on them and a worse stuffy nose will result when they are discontinued.

(429 words)

antibiotic /ˌæntɪbaɪˈɒtɪk/ *n.* 抗生素

allergic /əˈlɜːdʒɪk/ *adj.* 过敏的

bacterial /bækˈtɪərɪəl/ *adj.* 细菌的
complication /ˌkɒmplɪˈkeɪʃən/ *n.* 并发症
decongestant /ˌdiːkənˈdʒestənt/ *n.* 减充血剂
spray /spreɪ/ *n.* 喷雾

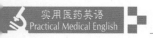

Text C

Pneumonia

Pneumonia is a lung infection which can result from a variety of causes, including infection with bacteria, viruses, fungi, or parasites, and chemical or physical injury to the lungs. Prior to the discovery of antibiotics, one-third of all people who developed pneumonia subsequently died from the infection. Today, pneumonia is still a leading cause of death among the elderly and people who are chronically and terminally ill.

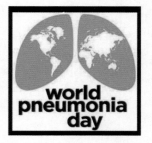

pneumonia /njuːˈməʊnɪə/
n. 肺炎
fungi /fʌŋdʒaɪ/
n.(fungus 的复数）真菌
parasite /ˈpærəsaɪt/
n. 寄生虫
subsequently
/ˈsʌbsɪkwəntli/
adv. 后来

Typical symptoms associated with pneumonia include a cough, chest pain, fever, and difficulty in breathing. People with infectious pneumonia often have a cough producing greenish or yellow sputum and a high fever that may be accompanied by shaking chills. Shortness of breath is also common. People with pneumonia may cough up blood, experience headaches, or develop sweaty and clammy skin. Other possible symptoms are the loss of appetite, fatigue, blueness of the skin, nausea, vomiting, mood swings, and joint pains or muscle aches.

accompany /əˈkʌmpəni/
vt. 伴随

clammy /ˈklæmi/
adj. 湿黏的
fatigue /fəˈtiːɡ/ n. 疲劳

To diagnose pneumonia health care providers rely on a patient's symptoms and findings from physical examination. Information from a chest X-ray, blood tests, and sputum cultures may also be helpful. The chest X-ray is typically used for diagnosis in hospitals and some clinics with X-ray facilities. Occasionally a chest CT scan or other tests may be needed to distinguish pneumonia from other illnesses.

culture /ˈkʌltʃə/
n.（细菌）培养

Most cases of pneumonia can be treated without hospitalization. Typically, oral antibiotics, rest, fluids, and home care are sufficient for complete resolution. However, people with pneumonia who are having trouble breathing, people with other medical problems, and the elderly may need more advanced treatment. If the symptoms get worse, the pneumonia does not improve with home treatment, or complications occur, the person will often have to be

hospitalization
/ˌhɒspɪtəlaɪˈzeɪʃən/
n. 住院治疗

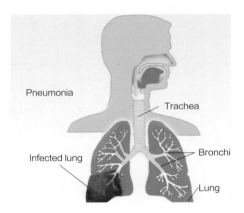

Pneumonia

Trachea

Bronchi

Infected lung

Lung

hospitalized.

Antibiotics are used to treat bacterial pneumonia. In contrast, antibiotics are not useful for viral pneumonia. The antibiotic choice depends on the nature of the pneumonia. Treatment for pneumonia should ideally be based on the causative microorganism and its known antibiotic sensitivity.

People who have difficulty breathing due to pneumonia may require extra oxygen. Extremely sick individuals may require intensive care treatment, often including intubation and artificial ventilation.

Sometimes pneumonia can lead to additional complications. Complications are more frequently associated with bacterial pneumonia than with viral pneumonia. The most important complications include: respiratory and circulatory failure, pleural effusion, emphysema, and abscess.

Nursing interventions and responsibilities in caring for the patient with pneumonia include administering oxygen and medications as prescribed and monitoring for their effects, monitoring vital signs, monitoring lung sounds, watching for edema and patients' feeling of shortness of breath. If the patient is immobile, it is imperative that the patient be turned every two hours and encouraged to cough and deep breathe.

(446 words)

microorganism
/ˌmaɪkrəʊˈɒːɡənɪzəm/
n. 微生物
sensitivity /ˌsensɪˈtɪvɪti/
n. 灵敏性
artificial /ˌɑːtɪˈfɪʃəl/
adj. 人工的
ventilation /ˌventɪˈleɪʃən/
n. 流通空气
pleural /ˈplʊərə/
adj. 胸膜的
effusion/ɪˈfjuːʒən/
n. 流出物
abscess /ˈæbses/
n. 脓肿
administer /ədˈmɪnɪstə/
vt. 给予
edema /ɪˈdiːmə/
n. 浮肿，水肿
imperative /ɪmˈperətɪv/
adj. 必要的

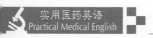

Exercises

Task 1   Oral Practice

Direction: Describe the common cold symptoms to your partner. You may use the
           following expressions for references.

under the weather

feel exhausted or fatigued

lack of energy

feel a headache, nausea and vomiting

feel light-headed

loss of appetite, weight loss, excessive fatigue, fever and chills

feel drowsy, dizzy and nauseated

have a persistent cough

cough up rusty or greenish-yellow phlegm

have a sore throat and a stuffy nose

have a fever, aching muscles and constant cough

cough with sputum and a feeling of malaise

have a headache, aching bones and joints

have bouts of uncontrollable coughing

have a runny nose, sneezing or a scratchy throat

have a stabbing pain that comes on suddenly in one or both temples

Task 2   Vocabulary Exercise

Direction: Match the words or phrases with similar meaning in the two columns.

A	B
1. contagious	a. necessary for living
2. organism	b. saliva
3. complication	c. growth of bacteria
4. vital	d. spreading by contact
5. nausea	e. new development of illness
6. culture	f. collection of pus formed in the body
7. bacterial	g. difficulty in breathing
8. abscess	h. living being
9. sputum	i. a feeling of sickness or disgust
10. dyspnea	j. of bacteria

Task 3　Reading Comprehension

Direction: Answer the following questions according to Text A and Text B.

1. Why is common cold a frequent and recurring problem?

2. What are the symptoms of a common cold?

3. What tests can be used to diagnose pneumonia?

4. What nursing interventions and responsibilities should be included in caring for the patient with pneumonia?

Task 4　Translation

Direction: Put the passage into Chinese with the help of your dictionary.

Symptoms of lower respiratory infections include a cough, fever, chest pain, tachypnea and sputum production. A cough is the typical initial presentation in acute bronchitis. Mucopurulent sputum may be present, and moderate temperature elevations occur. Typical findings in chronic bronchitis are an incessant cough and production of large amounts of sputum, particularly in the morning. Development of respiratory infections can lead to acute exacerbations of symptoms with possibly severe respiratory distress. Fever is common. A deepening cough, increased respiratory rate, and restlessness follow. Patients with pneumonia may also exhibit non-respiratory symptoms such as confusion, headache, myalgia, abdominal pain, nausea, vomiting and diarrhea.

Task 5　Prefixes, Suffixes and Roots

Direction: Learn the prefixes, suffixes or roots in the table and then choose the best answers.

Respiratory System (呼吸系统)

汉语 / 英语	常用词根	例词
呼吸 breath	-pnea pneum(o)- -spir(o)	tachypnea 呼吸过速；bradypnea 呼吸过缓； dyspnea 呼吸困难 pneumothorax 气胸 expiration 呼气；inspiration 吸气
鼻 nose	rhin(o)- naso-	rhinitis 鼻炎；rhinorrhoea 鼻漏 nasobronchial 鼻支气管；nasoscope 鼻镜； endonasopharyngeal 鼻咽内的
喉 larynx	laryng(o)-	laryngitis 喉炎；laryngectomy 喉切除术

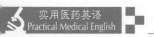
(Continued)

汉语 / 英语	常用词根	例词
咽 pharynx	pharyng(o)-	pharyngeal 咽部 pharyngitis 咽炎；pharyngoplasty 咽成形术；rhinopharynx 鼻咽
气管 windpipe	trache(o)-	tracheotomy 气管切开术；trachitis 气管炎；tracheobronchitis 气管支气管炎
支气管 bronchi	bronch(o)-	bronchiectasis 支气管扩张；bronchitis 支气管炎；bronchoscope 支气管镜；bronchogenic 支气管原的
肺 lung	pneumon(o)- pulmo(n)-	pneumonia 肺炎；bronchopneumonia 支气管肺炎 pulmonary 肺的；bronchopulmonary 支气管肺的
胸膜 pleura	pleur(o)-	pleuritis 胸膜炎；pleural 胸膜的

1. The word "windpipe" is related to _____.

    A. trachy-   B. trachelo-   C. teacho-   D. tracheo-

2. In medical term, the combining form strictly related to "larynx" is _____.

    A. laryngo-   B. larygo-   C. pharyngo-   D. pharygo-

3. Which word in the following has nothing to do with "breath"?

    A. Inspiration.   B. Spirochaeta.   C.Expiration.   D. Respiration.

4. The correct spelling for the word "支气管炎" is_____.

    A. bronchoitis   B. brancheitis   C. bronchitis   D. bronchoeitis

5. Which word in the following represents the abnormal respiration?

    A. Pneumoperitonue.   B. Orthopnea.

    C. Expiration.   D. Pneumaturia.

6. The combining form "spiro-" is related to _____.

    A. breath   B. air   C. lung   D. chest

7. The combining form only denoting relationship to "lung" is _____.

    A. pleur(o)-   B. pneumati-   C. pneumono-   D. alve(o)-

8. The English term for "气管切开术" is_____.

    A. tracheotomy   B. tracheoectomy   C. bronchiectomy   D. bronchoectomy

9. The word "breath" is not related to _____.

    A. pneum(o)-   B. pneumat(o)-   C. pneumon(o)-   D.-pnea

10. The expression for lung function which is used most often is _____.

    A. pneumonofunction   B. pneumofunction

    C. pulmonary function   D. pulmofunction

Task 6   Practical Writing

Direction: Read the following practical writing samples carefully and then write a similar application letter and design a medication template by yourself.

Sample 1

An Application Letter

May 10, 2017

Dear Mr. Wang,

How do you do? My name is Liu Fang, and I get the latest information from the local newspaper that you need some nurses. I am very interested in the job. So I am writing to you to apply for the nurse position in the surgical department of your hospital.

I graduated from the Nursing Department of Chongqing Medical College. After three years of work, including ten-month clinical practice in various departments in Southwest Hospital, I have acquired sound knowledge and core competencies of nursing. Besides, I worked as a volunteer in a gerocomium near our college and obtained some experience of caring for senior citizens. I passed the national exam for nurse license last year and worked as a registered nurse in a private clinic in the last half year. I am now confident that I am well prepared to be a qualified nurse in a general hospital like yours.

I enclose a resume, some copies of my qualifications and certificates, as well as a personal reference from my college teacher.

Thank you for reading my letter. I am looking forward to your reply.

Sincerely yours,

Liu Fang

Sample 2

A Medication Template

Sample medication template		
Patient name _____ Allergies _____ Healthcare provider _____ Phone number _____		
Medication (brand and generic names)	Dosage and frequency	Reason for use
--------------------------------		

UNIT THREE

Learning Objectives

After studying this unit, you will be able to:

- ❑ Enlarge your vocabulary related to a pharmacy and medical equipment;
- ❑ Talk about CPR;
- ❑ Know how to introducing the ward;
- ❑ Know how to admit a patient;
- ❑ Know something about SARS and flu;
- ❑ Know some prefixes, suffixes or roots of medical terms about circulatory system;
- ❑ Write a resume or a screening guideline overview.

Part 1   Pictures and Charts

Warming-up: Look at the following pictures, talk about them and then finish the task.

Picture 1

CPR

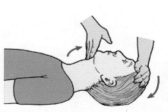 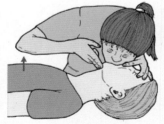

1. Tilt the head back and lift the chin until the teeth almost touch. Look and listen for breathing.

2. If the person is not breathing, pinch the nose closed and cover the person's mouth with yours. Give 2 full breaths.

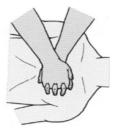 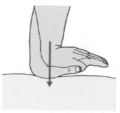

3. Put your hands in the center of the person's chest between the nipples. Place one hand on top of the other. Push down 30 times. Continue with 2 breaths then 30 pushes until medical help arrives or the person starts moving.

Picture 2

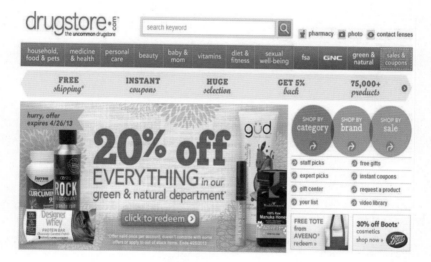

Picture 3

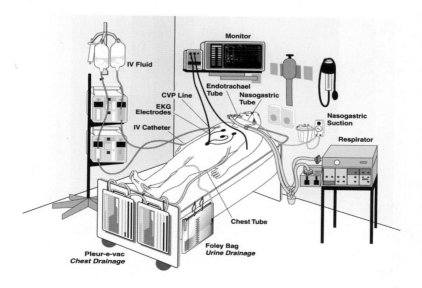

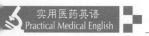
Task: Match the words in the left column with the explanations in the right column.

1. pharmacy	A. an apparatus used to provide artificial respiration
2. respirator	B. the process of removing air or liquid from a space or container, creating a partial vacuum that causes something else to be sucked in or surface to stick together
3. suction	C. a place where medicinal drugs are prepared or sold
4. catheter	D. a flexible tube inserted into the bladder or another body cavity, for removing fluid
5. drugstore	E. pharmacy

Part 2   Listening and Speaking

Conversation A

Introducing the Ward

(*Smallpox, a nurse, is receiving her patient, Burn.*)

Smallpox: How do you do？ Is this the first time you have been hospitalized, Mr. Burn？

Burn: Yes. I hope it's also the last time.

Smallpox: You will recover soon. I'm Smallpox, your duty nurse today. Please follow me and I'll show your bed.

Burn: Thank you.

hospitalize /ˈhɒspɪtlaɪz/
vt. 住院

Smallpox: Here is your bed. This is No.4 ward of the Internal Medicine Department. Your bed is number 25. Doctor Lee is responsible for your treatment. The call button is here.

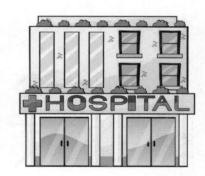

Burn: When should I use the call button？

Smallpox: You may press it if you need urgent help.

Burn: Thanks. What can I do with this bedside table？

Smallpox: You can put your change, toothbrush, toothpaste, towel, toilet paper and other daily necessities you need in the drawer

necessity /nɪˈsesɪti/
n. 必需品

of your bedside table.

Burn: Can I put my jewelry here?

Smallpox: No. If you have any valuables, deposit them in the safe in the nurses' office.

valuables /ˈvæljuəblz/
n. 贵重物品

Burn: Oh, I see. But, where is the toilet?

Smallpox: Just to the right of the door. If it is occupied, there is another one at the end of the passage on this floor.

Burn: When and where can I have my meals?

Smallpox: The hospital canteen downstairs is open twenty-four hours per day.

Burn: When are my relatives and friends allowed to visit me here?

Smallpox: Visitors are permitted here only from 3 p.m. to 5 p.m.

Burn: Thank you for all the information. You have made me feel at ease.

Smallpox: All the doctors and nurses here are kind and helpful. So, don't hesitate to ask us for help if you have any problems. We hope you have a good time here and recover very soon!

(292 words)

Conversation B

Admitting a Patient

Task 1: Watch episode one and fill in the missing words referring to the original text. Then check your writing against the original.

Nurse: Good morning, Mrs. Wilson. I am the nurse of the _____. My name is Emily. I'll be _____ you to the ward today.

Patient: Good morning, Emily. What should I do now?

Nurse: Would you please come with me to the nurses' office so I can finish the paperwork first?

Patient: Sure. May I sit down?

Nurse: Yes, of course. Please sit down and make yourself comfortable, OK? Can you tell me your full name and your date of birth?

Patient: My full name is Rose Wilson. And I was born on _____, 1968.

Nurse: Can you tell me why you are here today?

Patient: Well, um. I've had a duodenal ulcer for about five years. My _____ have been

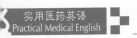

black for the past two days. I feel weak, too. My occult blood test is＿＿＿＿, so my doctor suggested I come here.

Task 2: Watch episode two and complete the answers according to the questions.

1. What causes Mrs. Wilson's duodenal ulcer?

It came from too much ＿＿＿＿ in her job.

2. What's the result of Mrs. Wilson's BP?

It's ＿＿＿＿＿.

3. Why does Mrs. Wilson think her pulse is too fast?

Because she always feels ＿＿＿＿＿these days.

Part 3　Reading Comprehension

Text A

CPR

If you've ever watched a hospital show on TV, you've probably seen *cardiopulmonary resuscitation*. It's called CPR for short and it saves lives. Let's find out how it works.

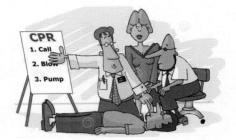

What Is CPR?

Cardio means "of the heart" and pulmonary means "of the lungs". Resuscitation is a medical word that means "to revive"—or bring back to life. Sometimes CPR can help a person who has stopped breathing, and whose heart may have stopped beating, to stay alive.

The person giving CPR—called a rescuer—follows three main steps, which are known as C-A-B:

C: do chest *compressions*

A: check the *airway*

B: do rescue *breathing*

compression /
kəmˈpreʃən/ *n.* 挤压

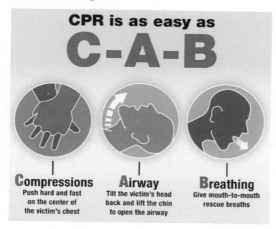

Chest Compressions

Someone giving CPR (the rescuer) will probably use both hands, one placed over the other, to press on the person's chest many times to move blood out of the heart that has stopped beating.

These are called chest compressions, and they help move oxygen-carrying blood to the body's vital organs—especially the all-important brain. A person who goes too long without oxygen reaching the brain will die.

vital /ˈvaɪtl/
adj. 至关重要的

In between each compression, the hands are lifted off the chest to let the chest go back to where it was. This allows blood to flow back toward the heart. In this way, the rescuer can keep the person alive by continuing to supply blood and oxygen to the brain and the rest of the body, until emergency help—like the paramedics—arrives to take the person to a hospital.

paramedic /pærəˈmedɪk/
n. 医护人员

Checking the Airways

After 30 compressions have been completed, the rescuer checks the airway to see if the person is breathing.

Rescue Breathing

If the person is not breathing, *two* rescue breaths are given. This is called artificial respiration. To do this, a rescuer puts his or her mouth over the other person's open mouth and blows, forcing

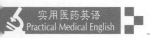
air into the lungs.(Ideally, the rescuer will use a special mask so that their mouths don't actually have to touch). Rescue breathing helps to move oxygen down into the lungs of the person who isn't breathing. Chest compressions should start again right after the two breaths are given.

When Should Someone Use CPR?

The steps in CPR (compressions, airway, and breathing) should be used whenever someone is not breathing and when the heart is not beating. If an emergency happens or someone becomes very sick while you're around, do your best to stay calm. First, try to get the person to respond by gently shaking his or her shoulder and asking,"Are you OK? " If there is no response and you are certified in CPR, you can begin CPR. If you're alone, and can't perform CPR, shout for help or call 120 by yourself.

certify /'sɜ:tɪfaɪ/
vt. 发证书给（某人）

Who Should Know CPR?

Certain people need to know how to perform CPR to do their jobs. Medical professionals— from nurses and doctors to paramedics and emergency medical technicians—must know CPR. Lifeguards, childcare workers, school coaches, and trainers usually have to learn CPR. Other adults who have family members with medical conditions such as heart disease sometimes know CPR, too.

(509 words)

Text B

Severe Acute Respiratory Syndrome

Severe acute respiratory syndrome (SARS) is a respiratory disease in humans which is caused by the SARS coronavirus (SARS-CoV). There has been one pandemic, between November 2002 and July 2003, with 8,090 known infected cases and 774 deaths (a mortality rate of 9.6%) worldwide being listed in the World Health Organization's (WHO) April 21, 2004 report.

coronavirus
/kɒrənə'vaɪrəs/
n. 冠状病毒
pandemic /pæn'demɪk/
n. 流行病
mortality /mɔ:'tæləti/
n. 死亡率

Cases of SARS in Some Countries or Regions

(1 November 2002—31 July 2003)

Country or Region	Cases	Deaths	Mortality(%)
Mainland China	5328	349	6.6
Hong Kong, China	1755	299	17
Canada	251	43	17
Taiwan,China	346	37	11
Singapore	238	33	14
Vietnam	63	5	8
USA	27	0	0
Philippines	14	2	14
Germany	9	0	0
Mongolia	9	0	0
Thailand	9	2	22
France	7	1	14
Malaysia	5	2	40
Sweden	5	0	0
Italy	4	0	0
UK	4	0	0
India	3	0	0
Republic of Korea	3	0	0
Indonesia	2	0	0
South Africa	1	1	100
Macau,China	1	0	0
Kuwait, Ireland, Romania Russian, Spain, Switzerland	Each has one case	0	0
Total	8090	774	9.6

(Adapted from the Source of WHO)

Initial symptoms are flu-like and may include: fever, myalgia, lethargy, gastrointestinal symptoms, cough, sore throat and other non-specific symptoms. The only symptom that is common to all patients appears to be a fever above 38℃. Shortness of breath

initial /ɪˈnɪʃəl/
adj. 最初的
myalgia /maɪˈældʒə/
n. 肌痛
lethargy /ˈleθədʒi/
n. 无生气
gastrointestinal
/ˌgæstrəʊɪnˈtestənl/
adj. 胃与肠的
syndrome /ˈsɪndrəʊm/
n. 症状

may occur later. Symptoms usually appear 2 to 10 days following exposure. However, up to 13 days has been reported. In most cases, symptoms appear within 2 to 3 days.

The Chest X-ray (CXR) appearance of SARS is variable. The initial CXR may be clear. White blood cell and platelet counts are often low.

platelet /'pleɪtlɪt/
n. 血小板

Antibiotics are ineffective as SARS is a viral disease. Treatment of SARS so far has been largely supportive with antipyretics, supplemental oxygen and ventilatory support as needed. Suspected cases of SARS must be isolated.

antipyretic /ˌæntɪpaɪ'retɪk/
n. 退热剂
supplemental /ˌsʌpli'mentl/
adj. 补足的
ventilatory /'ventɪlətərɪ/
adj. 通气的

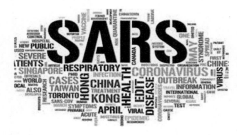

There was initially anecdotal support for steroids and the antiviral drug ribavirin, but no published evidence has supported this therapy. Many clinicians now suspect that ribavirin is detrimental. Researchers are currently testing all known antiviral treatments for other diseases including AIDS, hepatitis, influenza and others on the SARS-causing coronavirus.

anecdotal /ˌænik'dəutl/
adj. 传闻的
ribavirin /raɪbə'vaɪərɪn/
n. 病毒唑（抗病毒药）
clinician /klɪ'nɪʃən/
n. 临床医生
detrimental /ˌdetrɪ'mentl/
adj. 有害的
hepatitis /ˌhepə'taɪtɪs/
n. 肝炎
immune /ɪ'mju:n/
adj. 免疫的
modulate /'mɒdjʊleɪt/
vt. 调节

There is some evidence that some of the more serious damage in SARS is due to the body's own immune system overreacting to the virus. There may be some benefit from using steroids and other immune modulating agents in the treatment of the more acute SARS patients. Research is continuing in this area.

(420 words)

Text C

Bird Flu

Bird flu is also called avian flu, avian influenza, H5N1. "Bird flu" is a phrase similar to "swine flu", "dog flu", "horse flu", or "human flu" in that it refers to an illness caused by any of many different strains of influenza viruses that have adapted to a specific host.

avian /'eɪvɪən/
adj. 鸟类的 n. 鸟
influenza /ˌɪnflu'enzə/
n. 流行性感冒
host /həust/ n. 宿主

Birds, just like people, get the flu. Bird flu viruses infect birds, including chickens, ducks, other poultry and wild birds. However, bird flu can pose health risks to people. The first case of a bird flu virus infecting a person directly, H5N1, was in Hong Kong，China in 1997. Since then, the bird flu virus has spread to birds in countries in Asia, Africa and Europe.

poultry /ˈpəʊltri/
n. 家禽

Human infection is still very rare, but the virus that causes the infection in birds might change, or mutate, to more easily infect humans. This could lead to a pandemic or a worldwide outbreak of the illness.

mutate /mjuːˈteɪt/
vi. 变异

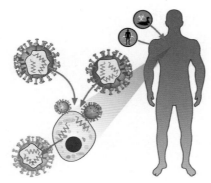

During an outbreak of bird flu, people who have contact with infected birds can become sick. It may also be possible to catch bird flu by eating poultry that is not well cooked or through contact with a person who has it. Bird flu can make people very sick or even cause death. There is currently no vaccine.

vaccine /ˈvæksiːn/
n. 疫苗
intestine /ɪnˈtestɪn/ n. 肠
domesticate
/dəˈmestɪkeɪt/
vt. 驯养（动物）
saliva /səˈlaɪvə/ n. 唾液
secretion /siˈkriːʃən/
n. 分泌物
feces/ˈfiːsiːz/
n. 粪便，排泄物
susceptible /səˈseptəbl/
adj. 易受影响的
contaminate
/kənˈtæmɪneɪt/ vt. 污染

Avian influenza viruses occur naturally among birds. Wild birds worldwide carry the viruses in their intestines, but usually do not get sick from them. However, avian influenza is very contagious among birds and can make some domesticated birds, including chickens, ducks and turkeys, very sick and kill them.

Infected birds shed influenza virus in their saliva, nasal secretions, and feces. Susceptible birds become infected when they have contact with contaminated secretions or excretions or with surfaces that are contaminated with secretions or excretions from infected birds. Domesticated birds may become infected with avian influenza virus through direct contact with infected waterfowl or other infected poultry, or through contact with surfaces (such as

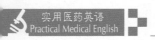
dirt or cages) or materials (such as water or feed) that have been contaminated with the virus.

feed /fi:d/ *n.* 饲料

Symptoms of avian influenza in humans have ranged from typical human influenza-like symptoms (e.g. fever, cough, sore throat, and muscle aches) to eye infections, pneumonia, severe respiratory diseases (such as acute respiratory distress), and other severe and life-threatening complications. The symptoms of avian influenza may depend on which virus caused the infection.

distress /dɪsˈtres/ *n.* 窘迫

Studies done in laboratories suggest that some of the prescription medicines should work in treating avian influenza infection in humans. However, influenza viruses can become resistant to these drugs, so these medications may not always work. Additional studies are needed to demonstrate the effectiveness of these medicines.

prescription /prɪˈskrɪpʃən/ *n.* 处方

resistant /rɪˈzɪstənt/ *adj.* 有耐药性的

(440 words)

Exercises

Task 1　Oral Practice

Direction: Study the following Chongqing Hot Pot menu and explain in English to your partner which system each organ belongs to.

Example: *Cow liver belongs to cow's digestive system.*

品名 Name	品名 Name
功夫牛肝 Kongfu Cow Liver	鲜肚条 Fresh Tripe
鲜鸭肠 Fresh Duck Intestine	鲜鱼肚 Fish Bladder
鲜牛鞭 Fresh Cow Penis	鸡肾 Chicken Kidney
无骨凤爪 Boneless Chicken Paw	牛黄喉 Cow Throat
鲜牛蹄筋 Fresh Cow Tendon	鲜脑花 Fresh Pig Brain

Task 2　Vocabulary Exercise

Direction: Match the words or phrases with similar meaning in the two columns.

A | B
1. isolate | a. death rate

2. hepatitis	b. muscle pain
3. mutate	c. to pollute
4. sore	d. a doctor's order for the use of a medicine
5. myalgia	e. live trouble
6. mortality	f. to change
7. host	g. to separate
8. prescription	h. aching
9. poultry	i. an animal or a plant on which a parasite lives
10. contaminate	j. domesticated birds

Task 3   Reading Comprehension

Direction: Decide whether the following statements are true or false according to Text A and Text B.

1. According to the World Health Organization's (WHO) report, in the pandemic of SARS between November 2002 and July 2003, the highest mortality rate occurred in Mainland China.

2. Fever, myalgia, lethargy, gastrointestinal symptoms, cough, sore throat, shortness of breath and other non-specific symptoms are the symptoms that are common to all SARS patients.

3. Antibiotics are ineffective as SARS is a viral disease. However, antipyretics are supposed to be useful in the treatment of SARS.

4. It is impossible to catch bird flu by eating poultry that is not well cooked or through contact with a person who has it.

5. Wild birds worldwide carry the viruses in their intestines, but usually do not get sick from them.

Task 4   Translation

Direction: Put the passage into Chinese with the help of your dictionary.

The main way that SARS seems to spread is by close person-to-person contact. The virus that causes SARS is thought to be transmitted most readily by respiratory droplets produced when an infected person coughs or sneezes. Droplet spread can happen when droplets from a cough or sneeze of an infected person are propelled a short distance (generally up to 3 feet) through the air and deposited on the mucous membranes of the mouth, nose, or eyes of those nearby. The virus also can spread

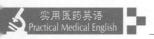

when a person touches a surface or object contaminated with infectious droplets and then touches his or her mouth, nose, or eye(s). In addition, it is possible that the SARS virus might spread more broadly through the air or by other ways that are not known yet.

Task 5   Prefixes, Suffixes and Roots

Direction: Learn the prefixes, suffixes or roots in the table and then choose the best answers.

Circulatory System（循环系统）

汉语/英语	常用词根	例　词
心 heart	cardi(o)- -cardium	electrocardiogram 心电图；carditis 心肌炎；phonocardiogram 心音图；cardiology 心（脏）病学 myocardium 心肌层；pericardium 心包膜
心房 atrium	atri/o-	atriotomy 心房切开术；periatrial 心房周的；transatrial 经心房的；atrial 心房的
心室 ventricle	ventricul-	supraventricular 室上的；ventriculocentesis 心室穿刺术；ventriculofiberscopy 心室纤维镜检查
瓣膜 valve	valvul(o)-	valvulitis 瓣膜炎；multivalvular 多瓣膜的；valvulopathy 心瓣病（valvectomy 瓣膜切除术）
血管 vessel	vas(o)- angi(o)-	vasculitis 血管炎；vasopressin 血管升压素 angiotensin 血管紧张素；angiography 血管造影
动脉 artery	arteri(o)-	arteriography 动脉造影术；arteritis 动脉炎；endoarteritis 动脉内膜炎；arteriosclerosis 动脉硬化
静脉 vein	ven(o)- phleb(o)-	venous 静脉的；intravenous 内静脉的 phlebitis 静脉炎；phlebography 静脉造影
脉搏 pulse	puls(o)-	pulseless 无脉的；pulsed 脉冲的

1. The Chinese meaning for the word "angiotensin" is _____.

　　A. 血管紧张素原　　B. 血管成型　　　　C. 血管舒缩活动　　D. 血管紧张素

2. The correct spelling for the word " 静脉造影 " is _____-graphy.

　　A. veino　　　　　B. arteri　　　　　C. vaso　　　　　D. phlebo

3. The combining form for the medical term " 心音图 " is phono-_____-gram.

　　A. heart　　　　　B. cardi　　　　　C. cardio　　　　D. cor

4. The Chinese explanation for "endoarteritis" is _____.

　　A. 动脉炎　　　　　B. 脉管炎　　　　　C. 动脉内膜炎　　　D. 主动脉炎

5. The English term for " 静脉炎 " is _____.

　　A. phlebitis　　　　B. veinitis　　　　　C. venitis　　　　D. venulitis

6. The word combining "arterio" with "graphy" means_____.

    A. 动脉成形术   B. 动脉造影术   C. 动脉石   D. 动脉内膜炎

7. To make a word about to the heart and blood vessels is _____.

    A. cardioventricular   B. cardioversion

    C. cardiovalvular   D. cardiovascular

8. Which word in the following means inflammation of the artery?

    A. Arteritis.   B. Atritis.   C. Arthritis.   D. Angitis.

9. The English equivalent for the word "血管炎" is _____.

    A. phlebitis   B. vessel inflammation

    C. vasculitis   D. angitis

10. Which form in the following has nothing to do with "脉搏"?

    A. pulse   B. impulse   C. pulso-   D. sphygmo-

Task 6   Practical Writing

Direction: Read the following practical writing samples carefully and then write a similar resume and design a screening guideline overview by yourself.

Sample 1

A Nurse's Resume

PERSONAL DETAILS

Name: Wang Fang   Address: 13, Bingjianglu, Wanzhou, Chongqing

Phone number: 135xxxxxxxx   E-mail address: wangfang@163.com

Date of Birth: May 12, 1980   Nationality: Chinese

EDUCATION DETAILS

Sept. 1997—July 2000 the Nursing Program, Chongqing Health School

Sept. 2001—July 2004 the Nursing Department, Chongqing Medical College

CAREER OBJECTIVES

I would like to gain further professional experience by working in a general hospital.

EMPLOYMENT HISTORY

13 November 2007—Present Xinhua Hospital

Registered Nurse   Full-time—40 hours per week   Position: Head Nurse

Responsibilities: This is a 283-bed hospital, with 8 theatres. I rotate in all areas of general surgery, orthopaedics, laparoscopic theatres, ENT, recovery and Gynaecology. The

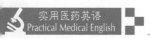

current roles and responsibilities involve clinical nursing, teaching and educational act as supervisor/mentor to all levels of staff both nursing and non-nursing. As a clinical nurse and team leader the responsibility involves assessment, planning, implementation and evaluation, maintaining patient and staff safety at all times within legislation guidelines and policies.

10 July 2005—6 Nov. 2007   Xiandai Hospital

Registered Nurse   Full-time—40 hours per week   Position: Nurse

Responsibilities: Working for a private hospital with 80 beds. A responsibility in the Emergency Department as a duty nurse involves work with up to 4 critically ill children, overseeing and caring for each patient.

PROFESSIONAL DEVELOPMENTS

1) Endoscopic Urology 1 week Course

2) Trauma Course

3) Fire and Safety

4) Basic Life Support

5) Legal Ethics Course

REFEREES

Name: Li Ping

Title: the director of Xinhua Hospital

Phone Number: 136xxxxxxxx

E-mail address: liping@sohu.com

Sample 2

Screening Guideline Overview

 Making the Difference . . . in School Health Screenings

	New Entrants	K	Gr.1	Gr.2	Gr.3	Gr.4	Gr.5	Gr.6	Gr.7	Gr.8	Gr.9	Gr.10	Gr.11	Gr.12
Scoliosis Screening							×	×	×	×	×			
Vision Screening														
Color Perception	×													
Near Vision	×													
Hyperopia	×													
Distance Acuity	×	×	×	×	×		×		×			×		
Hearing Screening	×	×	×		×		×		×			×		
Health Appraisals	×	×		×		×			×			×		

UNIT FOUR

Learning Objectives

After studying this unit, you will be able to:

- ❑ Enlarge your vocabulary related to the digestive system and common diseases;
- ❑ Talk about a physical exam;
- ❑ Practice a conversation taking place in the nurses' office;
- ❑ Know something about cerebral hemorrhage and diabetes;
- ❑ Know something about Traditional Chinese Medicine;
- ❑ Know some prefixes, suffixes or roots of medical terms about digestive system;
- ❑ Write a birth certificate and a flow sheet about the range of motion exercises.

Part 1   Pictures and Charts

Warming-up: Look at the following pictures, talk about them and then finish the task.

Picture 1

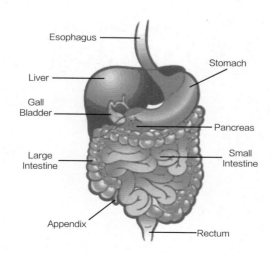

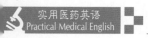

Picture 2

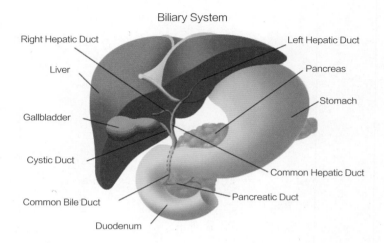

Picture 3

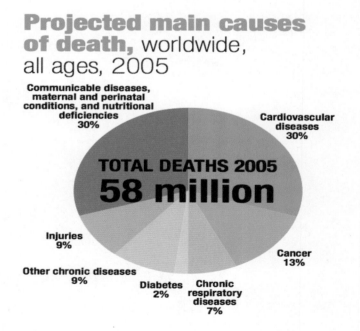

Task: Match the words in the left column with the explanations in the right column.

1. pancreas	A. the first part of the small intestine immediately beyond the stomach
2. duodenum	B. a large gland behind the stomach which produces digestive enzymes and release them into the duodenum
3. cancer	C. a lack or a weakness
4. chronic	D. a disease caused by an uncontrolled division of abnormal cells in a part of the body
5. deficiency	E. (of an illness or problem) lasting for a long time

Part 2   Listening and Speaking

Conversation A

Physical Examination

(A doctor is checking his patient.)

Doctor: Well, I am sorry you are ill. What's wrong with you?

Patient: Good morning, doctor. I feel dizzy.

Doctor: Have you had a fever?

Patient: No.

Doctor: Show me your tongue. Have you had any other symptoms such as a sore throat or a cough?

Patient: No, doctor.

Doctor: Have you been working very hard and felt very exhausted recently?

Patient: Recently, we have done a lot of tiring work.

Doctor: That's the reason. It's nothing serious, but you need to have a good rest for the next two to three days, and you will recover soon.

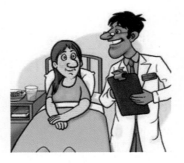

Patient: Thank you, doctor, but besides that, I have an upset stomach, too.

Doctor: How long ago did your stomach problems begin?

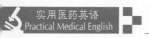
Patient: About three days ago.

Doctor: Do you feel nauseated?

Patient: No, not really.

Doctor: Have you vomited?

Patient: No.

Doctor: Is the pain regular?

Patient: Mm. I get pain quite often.

Doctor: Do you have any diarrhea?

Patient: Yes, a little bit. I usually have to go to the toilet when I have pain.

Doctor: How often do you have to go?

Patient: About four or five times a day.

Doctor: Have you had any trouble like this before?

Patient: It only happened when I was on business. I ate out a lot.

Doctor: Mm. Your general health is otherwise good?

Patient: Yes.

Doctor: And you're not taking any kind of medication regularly?

Patient: No.

Doctor: Well, this is simply diarrhea. It usually clears up in a few days. I'll just give you something for the diarrhea. Here's the prescription.

Patient: Thank you, doctor.

(273 words)

Conversation B

In the Nurses' Office

Task 1: Watch episode one and fill in the missing words referring to the original text. Then check your writing against the original.

Doctor: Hello. Mary, are you looking after Mr. John today?

Nurse: Yes. Any questions?

Doctor: Oh, can we take a few minutes to talk about his situation?

Nurse: Sure. Have a seat, please.

Doctor: Thank you. He was back from the OR an hour ago and there are a lot of orders for him. Let's make sure they are clear.

Nurse: Ok. Let me see._____, _____, _____every 30 minutes, temperature every 4 hours.
   And monitor the GCS every 4 hours.

Doctor: And also monitor his I & O, OK?

Nurse: Sure. How about his _____?

Doctor: Now his potassium levels are very low according to his blood result. Would you
   please give him a liter of Normal Saline with 20 millimoles of KCL?

Nurse: Sure. Please fill out the patient's _____ first.

Task 2: Watch episode two and complete the answers according to the questions.

1. How will the nurse run the antibiotics for Mr. John?

She will run them through a _____.

2. Besides antibiotics, what does the doctor want to give to Mr. John?

He wants to give him some _____with the fluids.

3. Why can these nutrients not be run through the cannula?

Because these nutrients are _____, and it's easy to cause _____.

Part 3   Reading Comprehension

Text A

Traditional Chinese Medicine

Chinese herbal medicine is one of the great herbal systems of the world, with an unbroken tradition going back to the 3rd century BC. Yet throughout its history it has continually developed in response to changing clinical conditions, and has been supported by research into every aspect of its use. This process continues today with the development of modern medical diagnostic techniques and knowledge.

herbal /'hɜːbl/
adj. 草药的

clinical /'klɪnɪkəl/
adj. 临床的

diagnostic /ˌdaɪəg'nɒstɪk/
adj. 诊断的

Because of its systematic approach and clinical effectiveness it has for centuries had a very great influence on the theory and practice of medicine in the East, and more recently has grown rapidly in popularity in the West. It still forms a major part of healthcare provision in China, and is provided in state hospitals alongside western medicine.

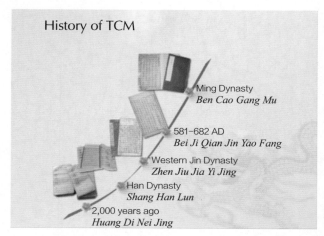

Chinese medicine includes all oriental traditions emerging from Southeast Asia that have their origins in China. Practitioners may work within a tradition that comes from Japan, Vietnam or Korea. It is a complete medical system that is capable of treating a very wide range of conditions. It includes herbal therapy, acupuncture, dietary therapy, and exercises in breathing and movement (Tai Chi and Qi Gong). Some or several of these may be employed in the course of treatment.

Chinese herbal medicine, along with the other components of Chinese medicine, is based on the concepts of Yin and Yang. It aims to understand and treat the many ways in which the fundamental balance and harmony between the two may be undermined and the ways in which a person's Qi or vitality may be depleted or blocked. Clinical strategies are based upon the diagnosis of patterns of signs and symptoms that reflect an imbalance.

vitality /vaɪˈtælɪti/
n. 生命力，活力
diagnosis /ˌdaɪəgˈnəʊsɪs/
n. 诊断

However, the tradition as a whole places great emphasis on lifestyle management in order to prevent disease before it occurs. Chinese medicine recognizes that health is more than just the absence of disease and it has a unique capacity to maintain and enhance our capacity for well being and happiness.

There is a growing body of research which indicates that traditional uses of plant remedies and the known pharmacological activity of plant constituents often coincide. However, herbal medicine is distinct from medicine based on pharmaceutical drugs.

remedy /remɪdi/ n. 疗法
pharmacological
/ˌfɑːməkəˈlɒdʒɪkəl/
adj. 药理学的

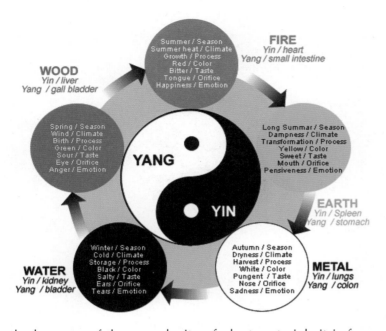

Firstly, because of the complexity of plant materials it is far more balanced than medicine based on isolated active ingredients and is far less likely to cause side effects. Secondly, because herbs are typically prescribed in combination, the different components of a formulae balance each other, and they undergo mutual coordination which increases efficacy and enhances safety. Thirdly, herbal medicine seeks primarily to correct internal imbalances rather than to treat symptoms alone, and therapeutic intervention is designed to encourage the body's self-healing process.

ingredient /ɪnˈgriːdiənt/ n. 成分

therapeutic /ˌθerəˈpjuːtɪk/ adj. 治疗的

(443 words)

Text B

Cerebral Hemorrhage

A cerebral hemorrhage is bleeding in the brain caused by the rupture of a blood vessel within the head.

Internal bleeding can occur in any part of the brain. Blood may accumulate in the brain tissues itself, or in the space between the brain and the membranes covering it. The bleeding may be isolated to part of one hemisphere or it may occur in other brain structures. An intracerebral hemorrhage can be caused by a traumatic brain

hemorrhage /ˈhemərɪdʒ/ n. 出血
rupture /ˈrʌptʃə/ n. 破裂
accumulate /əˈkjuːmjʊleɪt/ vi. 积聚
membrane /ˈmembreɪn/ n. 薄膜
hemisphere /ˈhemɪsfɪə/ n. 半球
intracerebral /ˌɪntrəˈserəbrəl/ adj. 大脑内的
traumatic /trɔːˈmætɪk/ adj. 创伤的

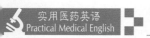

injury, brain tumours or abnormalities of the blood vessels. When it is not caused by one of these conditions, it is most commonly associated with high blood pressure. Blood irritates the brain tissues, causing swelling (cerebral edema). It can collect into a mass called a hematoma. Either swelling or a hematoma will increase pressure on brain tissues and can rapidly destroy them.

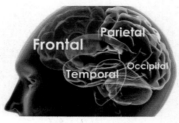

tumour /ˈtjuːmə/ n. 瘤
abnormality /ˌæbnɔːˈmælɪti/ n. 异常性
swelling /ˈswelɪŋ/ n. 肿胀
hematoma /hiːməˈtəumə/ n. 血肿

Symptoms vary depending on the location of the bleed and the amount of brain tissue affected. The symptoms usually develop suddenly, without warning, often during activities. It can cause headache, nausea, vomiting, changes in the level of consciousness, vision, sensation and movement, difficulty in speaking or understanding speech, swallowing, writing or reading, loss of coordination and balance.

nausea /ˈnɔːsiə/ n. 恶心
consciousness /ˈkɒnʃəsnɪs/ n. 意识

An intracerebral hemorrhage is a severe condition requiring prompt medical attention. It may develop quickly into a life-threatening situation. Treatment depends on the location, cause, and extent of the hemorrhage. Surgery may be needed, especially if there is bleeding in the cerebellum. Surgery may also be done to repair or remove structures causing the bleed. Medicines used may include painkillers, corticosteroids or diuretics to reduce swelling, and anticonvulsants to control seizures. Blood, blood products, and intravenous fluids may be needed to make up for loss of blood and fluids. Other treatments may be recommended, depending on the condition of the person and the symptoms that develop.

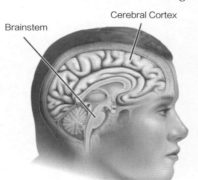

cerebellum /ˌserɪˈbeləm/ n. 小脑
corticosteroid /ˌkɔtɪkəuˈstɪərɒɪd/ n. 皮质类固醇
diuretic /ˌdaɪjuˈretɪk/ n. 利尿剂
anticonvulsant /ˌæntɪkənˈvʌlsənt/ n. 抗惊厥的药物
seizure /ˈsiːʒə/ n.（疾病）突然发作

How well a patient does depends on the size of the hematoma and the amount of swelling. Recovery may occur completely, or there may be some permanent loss of brain function. Death is possible, and may quickly occur despite prompt medical treatment. Medications, surgery, or other treatments may have severe side effects.

Treatment and control of underlying disorders may reduce the risk of developing intracerebral hemorrhage. High blood pressure should be treated. Do not stop taking medications unless told to do so by your doctor. Conditions such as an aneurysm can often be treated before they cause bleeding in the brain.

aneurysm /'ænjrɪzəm/
n. 动脉瘤

(405 words)

Text C

Diabetes Mellitus

Diabetes mellitus is a group of metabolic diseases characterized by high blood sugar (glucose) levels, which result from defects in insulin secretion, or action, or both.

diabetes /ˌdaɪə'biːtiːz/
n. 糖尿病
metabolic /ˌmetə'bɒlɪk/
adj. 新陈代谢的
glucose /'gluːkəus/
n. 葡萄糖
insulin /'ɪnsjulɪn/
n. 胰岛素
microvascular
/maɪkrəu'væskjulə/
adj. 微脉管的
atherosclerosis
/ˌæθərəusklɪ'rəusɪs/
n. 动脉硬化症
coronary /'kɒrənəri/
adj. 冠状的

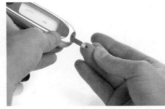

Diabetes can lead to blindness, kidney failure, and nerve damage. These types of damage are the result of damage to small vessels, referred to as a microvascular disease. Diabetes is also an important factor in accelerating the hardening and narrowing of the arteries (atherosclerosis), leading to strokes, coronary heart disease, and other large blood vessel diseases.

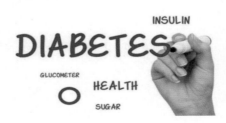

The early symptoms of untreated diabetes are related to elevated blood sugar levels, and loss of glucose in the urine. High amounts of glucose in the urine can cause increased urine output and lead to dehydration. Dehydration causes increased thirst and water consumption. The inability of insulin to perform normally has effects on protein, fat and carbohydrate metabolism. Insulin is an anabolic hormone, that is, one that encourages storage of fat and

dehydration
/ˌdiːhaɪ'dreɪʃən/ n. 脱水

hormone /'hɔː(r)məun/
n. 荷尔蒙，激素

protein. A relative or absolute insulin deficiency eventually leads to weight loss despite an increase in appetite. Some untreated diabetes patients also complain of fatigue, nausea and vomiting. Patients with diabetes are prone to develop infections of the bladder, skin, and vaginal areas. Fluctuations in blood glucose levels can lead to blurred vision. Extremely elevated glucose levels can lead to lethargy and coma.

vaginal /vəˈdʒaɪnəl/ *adj.* 阴道的
fluctuation /ˌflʌktʃʊˈeɪʃən/ *n.* 波动

Main Symptoms of Diabetes

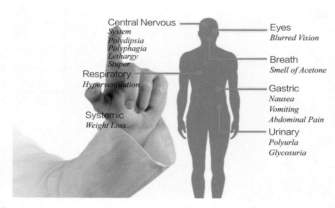

There are two major types of diabetes, called type 1 and type 2. Type 1 diabetes is also called insulin dependent diabetes mellitus (IDDM), or juvenile onset diabetes mellitus. In type 1 diabetes, the pancreas undergoes an autoimmune attack by the body itself, and is rendered incapable of making insulin. Type 2 diabetes is also referred to as non-insulin dependent diabetes mellitus (NIDDM), or adult onset diabetes mellitus (AODM). In type 2 diabetes, patients can still produce insulin, but do so relatively inadequately for their body's needs, particularly in the face of insulin resistance.

onset /ˈɒnset/ *n.* 发作
autoimmune /ˌɔːtəʊˈmjuːn/ *adj.* 自体免疫的

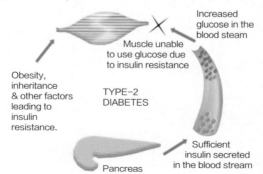

Aggressive and intensive control of elevated levels of blood sugar in patients with type 1 and type 2 diabetes decreases the complications of nephropathy, neuropathy, retinopathy, and may reduce the occurrence and severity of large blood vessel diseases. Aggressive control with intensive therapy means achieving fasting glucose levels between 70 to 120 mg/dl; glucose levels of less than 160 mg/dl after meals.

nephropathy /nəˈfrɒpəθɪ/ n. 肾病

neuropathy /njʊəˈrəpəθɪ/ n. 神经病

retinopathy /retɪˈnɒpəθɪ/ n. 视网膜病

fasting /ˈfɑːstɪŋ/ adj. 空腹的

The goal of diabetes management is to keep blood glucose levels as close to normal as safely possible. In addition, since diabetes may greatly increase a person's risk for heart disease, preventative measures for tightly controlling blood pressure and cholesterol levels are now an essential part of diabetes treatment as well.

cholesterol /kəˈlestərɒl/ n. 胆固醇

(423 words)

Exercises

Task 1   Oral Practice

Direction: You are asked to show some student nurses the techniques of giving an injection. Describe the steps and the important things which a nurse must pay attention to while he or she gives an injection. You can use the following words and expressions for reference.

intravenous injection	intramuscular injection	needle
1 milliliter	be allergic to	sterile procedure
push the syringe	cross infection	skin test dosage

Task 2   Vocabulary Exercise

Direction: Match the word with its Chinese meaning in the two columns.

A	B
1. hardening	a. 冠状的
2. rupture	b. 畸形
3. coronary	c. 组织
4. abnormality	d. 胰岛素
5. cerebellum	e. 淬水

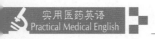

6. glucose   f. 波动

7. tissue   g. 破裂

8. insulin   h. 小脑

9. traumatic   i. 葡萄糖

10. fluctuation   j. 外伤的

Task 3　Reading Comprehension

Direction: Answer the following questions according to Text A and Text B.

1. What are the causes of cerebral hemorrhage?

2. What are the symptoms of cerebral hemorrhage?

3. What are the two types of diabetes mellitus?

4. How is diabetes treated?

Task 4　Translation

Direction: put the passage into Chinese with the help of your dictionary.

Juvenile diabetes is an autoimmune disorder which can be due to environmental trigger or virus, which hampers the function of the beta cell. Once the beta cells are destroyed, the body is unable to produce insulin. A child with diabetic siblings is more prone to develop juvenile diabetes than the child from a totally unaffected family. It is considered to be a more hereditary problem than excess eating or being obese. When your child is diagnosed with diabetes, it's easy to feel overwhelmed by all the information you're given. Managing diabetes is a matter of juggling three things: insulin, food and exercise. All three have a major effect on diabetes control.

Task 5　Prefixes, Suffixes and Roots

Direction: Learn the prefixes, suffixes or roots in the table and then choose the best
           answers.

Digestive System (消化系统)

汉语 / 英语	常用词根	例　词
食管 esophagus	esophag(o)-	esophagoscope 食管镜；gastroesophageal 胃食管的

(Continued)

汉语 / 英语	常用词根	例　词
胃 stomach	gastr(o)-; stomach(o)-	gastritis 胃炎；gastroscopy 胃镜检查；gastropathy 胃病 stomachache 胃痛
肠 intestine	enter(o)-	enteritis 肠炎；enterovirus 肠道病毒；enterobacteria 肠 道菌；gastroenteritis 胃肠炎
十二指肠 duodenum	duoden(o)-	duodenal 十二指肠的；gastroduodenal 胃十二指肠
结肠 colon	col(o)-; colon(o)-	colocentesis 结肠穿刺术；colitis 结肠炎；paracolic 结 肠周围的；colonoscopy 结肠镜检查
消化 digestion	peps(o)- -gest(o)-	dyspepsia 消化不良；pepsin 胃蛋白酶 digestive 消化的；digestible 可消化的
直肠 rectum	rect(o)- procto-	rectocele 直肠膨出；rectouterine 直肠子宫 proctoptosis 直肠脱垂；proctoscopy 直肠镜检查
胆囊 gallbladder; cholecyst	cholecyst(o)-	cholecystitis 胆囊炎；cholecystolithiasis/ cholelithiasis 胆囊结石病（或胆石症）
肝 liver	hepat(o)-	hepatitis 肝炎；hepatorrhexis 肝破裂
胆管 bile duct	cholangi(o)-	cholangitis 胆管炎；cholangiography 胆管造影术
阑尾 appendix	appendic(o)-	appendicitis 阑尾炎；appendicectomy 阑尾切除术

1. The Chinese meaning for "pepsin" is _____.

    A. 胃蛋白酶   B. 胃泌素   C. 胃蛋白酶原   D. 胃酶抑素

2. Fill in the blank with the combining part for the medical term "结肠镜检查":

    _____-scopy.

    A. entero   B. recto   C. colono   D. colo

3. The Chinese meaning for "cholecystitis" is_____.

    A. 胆囊炎   B. 膀胱炎   C. 肝炎   D. 胆管炎

4. The English term for "直肠脱垂" is _____.

    A. rectouterine   B. proctoptosis   C. colitis   D. rectocele

5. The term "duodenum" is so called because it is about twelve_____.

    A. fingerlengths   B. fingerbreadths

    C. fingercircle   D. fingercircumferrence

6. The word which has nothing to do with liver is _____.

    A. hepatitis   B. hepatolithiasis   C. hepatorrhexis   D. pancreatitis

7. The correct spelling for the word "胆管造影术" is _____.

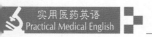

A. cholangiopancreatography   B. cholangiocarcinoma

C. cholangiography   D. cholecystectomy

8. The following words have the meaning of inflammation except_____.

    A. pancreatitis   B. hepatitis   C. cholangitis   D. gastropathy

9. Which word has the meaning of "胆囊切除术"?

    A. Hepatolithiasis.   B. Cholecystectomy.

    C. Cholecystolithiasis.   D. Cholecystotomy.

10. Which word has nothing to do with the stomach?

    A. Gastritis.   B. Gastropathy.   C. Stomatitis.   D. Stomachache.

Task 6   Practical Writing

Direction: Read the following practical writing samples carefully and fill in the blanks of the birth certificate with appropriate information. Then design a similar flow sheet about the range of motion exercises.

Sample 1

Birth Certificate

Full name of baby _____	Male ☐ Female ☐	Date of birth Year_____ Month_____ Day_____ Hour_____ Minute_____	
Place of birth _____	Province_____ City _____ Country (District)_____ Township_____		Gestation (week) _____ Weeks
Full name of mother _____		Age _____	Nationality _____
Identity card No. _____			
Full name of father _____		Age _____	Nationality _____
Identity card No. _____			
Type of place	General hospital ☐ MCH hospital ☐ Home ☐ Other ☐		
Name of facility_____			
Birth certificate No. _____		Date of issue Year _____ Month_____ Day_____	

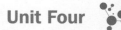

Sample 2

Range of Motion Exercises

FLOW SHEET—RANGE OF MOTION EXERCISES

Patient _____

Ward/Room/Bed/ _____ Date _____

MOVEMENT	TIME			COMMENTS
	0600	1700		
R Upper Extremity				
Shoulder flexion	√			
Shoulder external rotation	√			
Elbow extension	√			limited to 120
Wrist extension	√			
Finger extension	√			
R Lower Extremity				
Hip abduction	√			
Hip extension	√			
Knee extension	√			
Ankle dorsiflexion	√			
NURSE'S INITIALS	JHS			

UNIT FIVE

Learning Objectives

After studying this unit, you will be able to:

- ❑ Enlarge your vocabulary related to the digestive system;
- ❑ Know how to collect medical history in English;
- ❑ Know how to administer medications;
- ❑ Know something about leaflets on medical equipment use;
- ❑ Know something about CT and peptic ulcer;
- ❑ Know some prefixes, suffixes or roots of medical terms about urinary system;
- ❑ Write a certificate of sick leave and a certificate of discharge.

Part 1 Pictures and Charts

Warming-up: Look at the following pictures, talk about them and then finish the task.

Picture 1

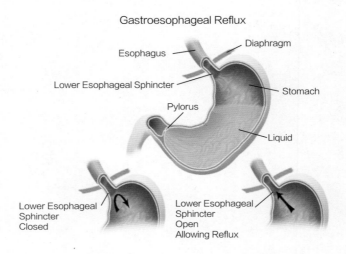

Picture 2

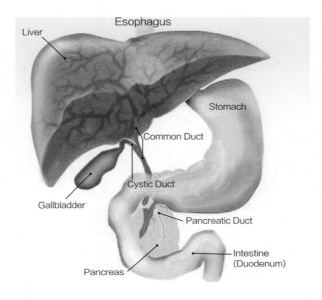

Esophagus

Liver

Stomach

Common Duct

Cystic Duct

Gallbladder

Pancreatic Duct

Intestine
(Duodenum)

Pancreas

Picture 3

How to Use
Easy, User-friendly Instruction

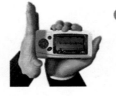

Method I
1 Turn on power and
place chest electrode
againts your left palm.

Method II
1 Place the chest
electrode on bare skin
about 5 cm (2 inch)
below your left nipple.

2 Keep the same posture
until measurement is
complete. It takes
about 30 seconds.

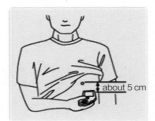

about 5 cm

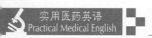

Task: Match the words in the left column with the explanations in the right column.

1. esophagus	A. the muscular tube which connects the throat to the stomach
2. pylorus	B. a tube in the body through which fluid passes
3. sphincter	C. the opening from the stomach into the small intestine
4. electrode	D. a conductor through which electricity enters or leaves something
5. duct	E. a ring of muscle that surrounds an opening such as the anus, and can be tightened to close it

Part 2   Listening and Speaking

Conversation A

Collecting Medical History

(The doctor is asking for the medical history of a patient.)

Doctor: Good Morning, Mr. Smith. What brings you here today?

Patient: Well, I've been having terrible headaches.

Doctor: When did they start?

Patient: Just a week ago.

Doctor: Could you tell me something more about your headache? What is the location of the pain? I mean, in which part of your head?

Patient: All over the forehead.

Doctor: How long do they last?

Patient: About an hour every time. Then, they just seem to disappear by themselves.

Doctor: Have you noticed that your vision has deteriorated recently?

delicacy /ˈdelɪkəsi/ *n.* 佳肴

Patient: Maybe. When I read books, the words sometimes seem blurred.

Doctor: Have you consulted a doctor lately?

Patient: No. The last time I did was about four years ago.

Doctor: Do you have trouble climbing steps or running fast?

Patient: Well, yes. Sometimes I have to stop and catch my breath.

Doctor: Do you ever have to get up at night to pass water?

Patient: Not very often.

Doctor: Have you had any swelling of your ankles?

Patient: No, I don't think so.

Doctor: Has anyone in your family ever had heart disease?

Patient: Yes. My mother died of high blood pressure.

Doctor: Have you always been this heavy?

Patient: Oh, Doctor, am I really heavy? My weight is just 90 kilograms.

Doctor: Just a bit overweight. Or, let's say you have a good appetite. What kind of food do you often eat?

Patient: Meat is my favorite. I have a lot of meat in every meal: pork, beef, and mutton, anything like that. No meal without meat for me!

Doctor: Losing some weight wouldn't hurt you.

Patient: I have been trying to be on a diet for many years, but each time I can't resist the temptation of the delicacies. So, I just put on more weight.

Doctor: All right, Mr. Smith. Would you please follow me to the examining room? I'd like to give you a physical exam.

temptation /temp'teɪʃən/ n. 诱惑

deteriorate /dɪ'tɪəriəreɪt/ v.(使) 恶化

(329 words)

Conversation B

Administering Medications

Task 1: Watch episode one and fill in the missing words referring to the original text. Then check your writing against the original.

Nurse: Hi, Janice, Good to see you again.

Patient: Thank you and me too. You look so nice today.

Nurse: How are you doing today?

Patient: Not good, I have a _____ and feel _____ today. My blood pressure was one eighty over one ten (180/110) this morning. That's really high, isn't it?

Nurse: Oh, I see. That's the reason why Dr. Peter _____ two new medications for you. One

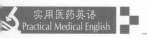
is Metoprolol, to _____ your BP. And another is Lasix, a diuretic.

Patient: Oh, I can't remember the names. Would you please repeat them?

Nurse: Sure, and I'll tell more about them. Metoprolol is in the green box, and I already wrote down the _____ for you. You take these 2 pills once, twice a day, that's 8 a.m. before your breakfast and 8 p.m. before your bedtime. Got it?

Patient: Mm, but I have a very poor memory. Instructions on the box are good for me.

Task 2: Watch episode two and complete the answers according to the questions.

1. Why should the patient put this medicine in a cool place?

Because it would be _____ at 45° C.

2. What's the function of Lasix?

It prevents our body from _____ too much _____.

3. What's the nurse's suggestion for diet?

The patient would better eat diet with more _____.

Part 3 Reading Comprehension

Text A

CT

You may be asked to fast for up to 4 hours prior to your scan. For scans of the abdomen and pelvis, the bowel needs to be opacified prior to the scan. This is done by drinking a barium or iodine-based dye prior to the scan. This usually takes 10 minutes or 1 to 2 hours, sometimes even 12 hours before the scan. No other special preparation is usually needed, but for some pelvic scans a small enema may be given immediately before the scan, and for some gynecological scans a tampon may be required.

In the scan room, you will lie on a table that subsequently moves slowly through a hole in the center of the scanner. You may require an intravenous injection of an iodine-based dye, or contrast agent during the scan. This circulates through your bloodstream, highlighting many organs and making abnormalities more conspicuous.

opacify /əʊˈpæsɪfaɪ/ vt. 使……变得不透明
barium /ˈbeərɪəm/ n. 钡
dye /daɪ/ n. 碘剂
enema /ˈenɪmə/ n. 灌肠剂
gynecological /ˌgaɪnəkəˈlɒdʒɪkəl/ adj. 妇产科的
intravenous /ˌɪntrəˈviːnəs/ adj. 通过静脉的
contrast agent 造影剂
conspicuous /kənˈspɪkjʊəs/ adj. 显著的

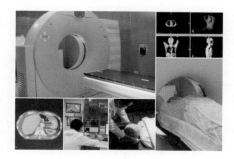

The dye is rapidly removed from the body by the kidneys. It is common to notice a warm sensation or a metallic taste in the mouth; these sensations pass quickly. Nausea, vomiting and allergic reactions to the dye are uncommon. People with impaired kidney function may not be able to receive the dye injection, and diabetics taking glucophage should have had a recent blood test for kidney function.

The dye is injected into a vein, usually at the elbow or wrist. It may be given as a hand injection by the doctor prior to the scan, or by an injection pump during the scan. During the scan the X-ray tube rotates around you; you will not see this as it is hidden by the scanner housing. You may be required to hold your breath during the scan. A typical scan takes 20 seconds to 2 minutes, depending on the type of scan you are having, although you should allow up to 30 minutes to include the setup time and time to print and check the images afterwards.

The images will be printed and the radiologist will study them and issue a report. The report is usually available to the referring doctor within 24 hours, or immediately in urgent cases.

(356 words)

Text B

Peptic Ulcer

Gastric ulcers or peptic ulcers are holes in the lining of the stomach and duodenum, usually caused by a bacterial infection of Helicobacter pylori (*H. pylori*). The stomach produces hydrochloric acid and enzymes, including pepsin, that break down and digest

---

Glossary (margin):

sensation /sen'seɪʃən/ *n.* 感觉

impaired /ɪm'peəd/ *adj.* 受损的

glucophage /'gluːkəʊfeɪdʒ/ *n.* 盐酸二甲双胍

rotate /rəʊ'teɪt/ *vi.* 旋转

radiologist /ˌreɪdi'ɒlədʒɪst/ *n.* 放射医师

duodenum /ˌdjuːə'diːnəm/ *n.* 十二指肠
Helicobacter pylori 幽门螺旋杆菌
hydrochloric acid /ˌhaɪdrə'klɒrɪk 'æsɪd/ 氢氯酸，盐酸
enzyme /'enzaɪm/ *n.* 酶
pepsin /'pepsɪn/ *n.* 胃蛋白酶

food. A mucous layer coats the stomach and protects it from the acid. Prostaglandins also aid in protecting the lining. When these defenses are not performing their job properly, acid and pepsin eat away at the lining, forming an open sore called an ulcer. *H. pylori* is an unease-enzyme-producing bacterium that decreases the stomach's ability to produce mucous, making it prone to acid-damage and peptic ulcers. Although *H. pylori* infection is found in many people, it does not cause ulcers in all of them. Not all ulcers are caused by these bacteria. Long-term use of no steroid anti-inflammatory agents (NSAIDs), such as aspirin, naproxen, and ibuprofen can also cause peptic ulcers.

mucous /'mju:kəs/
adj. 黏液的
prostaglandin
/ˌprɒstə'glændɪŋ/
n. 前列腺素
bacterium /bæk'tɪərɪəm/
n. 细菌（复数为 bacteria)
prone /prəʊn/ *adj.* 倾向于

steroid /'stɪərɒɪd/
n. 类固醇
naproxen /nə'prɒksɪn/
n. 萘普生
ibuprofen /ˌaɪbju:'prəʊfen/
n. 布洛芬

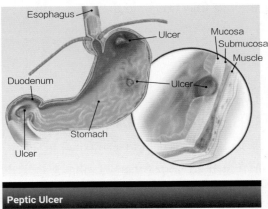

Peptic Ulcer

The most common symptom of duodenum ulcer is abdominal pain that is dull, comes and goes over a period of time, may occur a few hours after eating or during the night, and is relieved by food and antacids. Weight loss, bloating and nausea are lesser indicators. Symptoms that require immediate medical attention include sharp, sudden, persistent stomach pain, bloody or black stools, or bloody vomit or vomit that looks like coffee grounds.

antacid /ænt'æsɪd/
n. 抗酸剂
bloat /bləʊt/ *vi.* 膨胀
indicator /'ɪndɪkeɪtə/
n. 指示物

The laboratory diagnosis of peptic ulcers caused by *H. pylori* can be performed using a variety of different methods and specimen types. The most common laboratory test for diagnosing peptic ulcers is a blood test for the presence of antibodies to *H. pylori*. The presence of *H. pylori* antibodies means you have been infected at some time with this organism. A stool sample may be collected to look for the *H. pylori* antigen; however, this test is not appropriate

specimen /'spesɪmɪn/
n. 样本

organism /'ɔ:gənɪzəm/
n. 生物体，有机体
antigen /'æntɪdʒən/
n. 抗原

for individuals who have blood in their stool. A breath test is also available that detects the enzyme activity of *H. pylori*. Some invasive procedures may be used to diagnose an ulcer. These include an upper GI (gastrointestinal) series that involves taking x-rays of the GI tract and endoscopy, in which a tiny camera on the end of a thin tube is fed through the mouth, down the esophagus, to the duodenum.

endoscopy /enˈdɒskəpi/ *n.* 内窥镜检查法
esophagus /iːˈsɒfəgəs/ *n.* 食道（oesophagus 的美式拼法）

Peptic ulcers are rarely fatal, but if they penetrate the stomach or duodenal wall (perforation), break a blood vessel (hemorrhage), or block food leaving the stomach (obstruction), they can be very serious. Treatment usually involves a combination of antibiotics to kill the bacteria and drugs to reduce the amount of stomach acid produced.

penetrate /ˈpenɪtreɪt/ *vt.* 穿透
perforation /pɜːfəˈreɪʃən/ *n.* 穿孔

(427 words)

Text C

Acute Kidney Failure

Acute kidney failure is the sudden loss of your kidneys' ability to perform their main function—eliminate excess fluid and waste material from your blood. When your kidneys lose their filtering ability, dangerous levels of fluid and waste accumulate in your body.

eliminate /ɪˈlɪmɪneɪt/ *vt.* 排除

Acute kidney failure is most common in people who are already hospitalized, particularly people who need intensive care. Acute kidney failure tends to occur after complicated surgery, after a severe injury or when blood flow to your kidneys is disrupted.

disrupt /dɪsˈrʌpt/ *vt.* 使中断

Loss of kidney function may also develop gradually over time, with few signs or symptoms in the early stages. In this case, it's referred to as chronic kidney failure. High blood pressure and diabetes are the most common causes of chronic kidney failure.

Acute kidney failure can be serious and generally requires intensive treatment. Unlike the chronic form, however, acute kidney failure is reversible and if you're otherwise in good health you

reversible /rɪˈvɜːsəbl/ *adj.* 可逆的

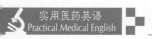
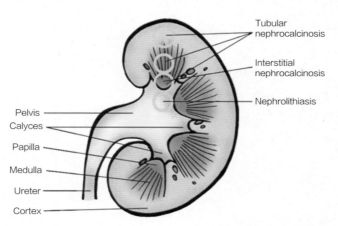

should recover normal kidney function within a few weeks. If acute kidney failure occurs in the context of severe chronic illness—a heart attack, stroke, overwhelming infection—the outcome is often worse.

overwhelming
/ˌəʊvəˈwelmɪŋ/
adj. 无法抵抗的

Signs and symptoms of acute kidney failure may include:

• Decreased urine output, although occasionally urine output remains normal;

• Fluid retention, causing swelling in your legs, ankles or feet;

retention /rɪˈtenʃən/
n. 潴留

• Drowsiness;

• Shortness of breath;

• Fatigue;

• Confusion;

• Seizures or coma in severe cases;

• Chest pain related to pericarditis, an inflammation of the saclike membrane that envelops your heart.

pericarditis
/ˌperɪkɑːˈdaɪtɪs/
n. 心包炎
inflammation
/ˌɪnfləˈmeɪʃən/ n. 炎症
envelop /ɪnˈveləp/
vt. 包围

Some people don't notice any early signs or symptoms, or are more bothered by the underlying problem causing sudden kidney failure.

Your kidneys are two bean-shaped organs, each about the size of your fist. They're located at the back of your upper abdomen, one on either side of your spine. Your kidneys are part of a system that removes excess fluid and waste material from your blood. Initially, blood enters your kidneys through the renal arteries, which are branches of the aorta—the main artery carrying oxygenated blood from your heart to the rest of your body. From there, blood moves

spine /spaɪn/
n. 脊柱，脊椎

aorta /eɪˈɔːtə/ n. 大动脉
oxygenate /ˈɒksɪdʒəneɪt/
vt. 氧化

through structures in your kidneys known as nephrons.

Each kidney contains approximately 1 million nephrons, each consisting of a tuft of capillary blood vessels (glomerulus) and tiny tubules that lead into larger collecting tubes. Each tuft of capillaries filters fluid from your bloodstream.

The filtered material, which contains both waste products and substances vital for your health, passes into the tubules. From there, waste byproducts—urea, uric acid and creatinine—are excreted in your urine, while substances your body needs—sugar, amino acids, calcium and salts—are reabsorbed back into your bloodstream.

(445 words)

nephron /'nefrɒn/
n. 肾单位，肾元
tuft /tʌft/ n. 一簇
capillary /kə'pɪləri/
n. 毛细血管
glomerulus
/gləʊ'meərjʊləs/
n.（肾）小球
tubule/'tjuːbjuːl/
n. 小管，细管
urea /jʊ'riːə/ n. 尿素
uric /'jʊərɪk/ adj. 尿的
creatinine /kriː'ætɪniːn/
n. 肌氨酸酐
amino /ə'miːnəʊ/
adj. 氨基的

Exercises

Task 1　Oral Practice

Direction: Explain in English what medical services the following medical personnel can offer.

Example：

a midwife engages in assisting in childbirth or providing antenatal, postnatal and neonatal care

1. midwife
2. physician
3. head nurse
4. pediatrician
5. gynecologist
6. obstetrician
7. neurologist
8. psychiatrist
9. oculist
10. dentist
11. surgeon
12. anesthetist

Task 2　Vocabulary Exercise

Direction: Match the words with similar meanings in the two columns.

A	B
1. peptic ulcers	a. a tuft of capillary blood vessels as nephrons in the kidney
2. Helicobacter pylori	b. the action of obstructing or the state of being obstructed
3. perforation	c. flow in the blood vessel
4. hemorrhage	d. exceed the range of natural blood pressure

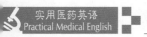
5. obstruction   e. a urease-enzyme-producing bacterium

6. glomerulus   f. holes in the lining of the stomach and duodenum

7. high blood pressure   g. a rapid loss of blood

8. bloodstream   h. penetration of the stomach or duodenal wall

Task 3　Reading Comprehension

Direction: Answer the following questions according to Text A and Text B.

1. Where do peptic ulcers happen?

2. What are the symptoms of acute kidney failure?

3. What tests can be used to diagnose peptic ulcers?

4. What nursing interventions and responsibilities should be included in caring for the patient with acute kidney failure?

Task 4　Translation

Direction: Put the passage into Chinese with the help of your dictionary.

    H. pylori lives and multiplies within the mucous layer that covers and protects tissues that line the stomach and small intestine. Often, H. pylori causes no problems. But sometimes it can disrupt the mucous layer and inflame the lining of the stomach or duodenum, producing an ulcer. One reason may be that people who develop peptic ulcers already have damage to the lining of the stomach or small intestine, making it easier for bacteria to invade and inflame tissues.

Task 5　Prefixes, Suffixes and Roots

Direction: Learn the prefixes, suffixes or roots in the table and then choose the best answers.

Urinary System (泌尿系统)

汉语 / 英语	常用词根	例　词
尿 urine	urin(o)- ur(o)-	urinary 尿的；urinogenital 泌尿生殖的 hematuria 血尿；polyuria 多尿症
肾 kidney	ren(o)- nephr(o)-	renovascular 肾血管的；suprarenal 肾上的 nephritis 肾炎；hydronephrosis 肾积水
膀胱 bladder	vesic(o)- cyst(o)-	vesical 膀胱的；rectovesical 直肠膀胱的 cystitis 膀胱炎；cystostomy 膀胱造瘘术

(Continued)

汉语 / 英语	常用词根	例　词
尿道 urethra	urethr(o)-; meat(o)-	urethritis 尿道炎；　urethroscopy 尿道镜检查 meatotomy 尿道口切开术；meatorrhaphy 尿道口缝合术
睾丸 testis	test(o)- testicul(o)- orchi(o)- didym(o)-	testosterone 睾酮 testicular 睾丸的 orchitis 睾丸炎 epididymis 附睾
前列腺 prostate	prostat(o)-	prostatic 前列腺的；prostatitis 前列腺炎；prostatectomy 前列腺切除术；prostatalgia 前列腺痛
肾盂 renal pelvis	pelvi(o)- pyel(o)-	pelvioplasty 肾盂造影术 pyelonephritis 肾盂肾炎；pyelography 肾盂造影术

1. Fill in the blank with the combining part for the medical term "尿道造影术"：_____
   -graphy.

    A. urino   B. ureter   C. urethro   D. urethra

2. The correct spelling for the word "尿道炎" is _____.

    A. uteritis   B. urinitis   C. ureteritis   D. urethritis

3. The correct spelling for the word "肾积水" is _____.

    A. hydrorenosis   B. hydronephrosis   C. hydrorenitis   D. hydronephritis

4. The word with Chinese meaning as "血尿" is _____.

    A. hematuria   B. hemaurine   C. hemaurinati   D. hemaurinary

5. Inflammation of the prostate is given the term as _____.

    A. orchitis   B. orchotitis   C. prostatitis   D. prostatotitis

6. Which word in the following has the meaning of "no urine"?

    A. Anuria.   B. Polyuria.   C. Anurine.   D. Polyurine.

7. Inflammation of the testis is given the term as _____.

    A. epididymoorchitis   B. orchitis

    C. epididymitis   D.epididymis

8. Fill in the blank with the combining part for the medical term "膀胱造影术"：_____
   -graphy.

    A. gall bladder   B. bladder   C. vesico   D. cysto

9. Which prefix in the following has nothing to do with "睾丸"?

    A. testiculo-   B. testo-   C. cysto-   D. orchi-

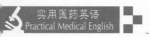
10. The correct spelling for the word "膀胱输尿管的" is _____.

    A. cystocoureteral   B. vesicoureteral

    C. vesicourethral   D. bladderureteral

Task 6　Practical Writing

Direction: Read the following practical writing samples carefully and then write similar certificates by yourself.

Sample 1

Certificate for Sick Leave

April 20, 2017

    This is to certify…, male, 25, has a high fever of 49 ℃ and a very serious sore throat. We advise that he should take a two-day rest, and if necessary, come back for a check in two days.

(Doctor's Signature)

Sample 2

Certificate of Discharge

May 25, 2017

    This is to certify that Mr. John Smith admitted on May 5, 2017 has had acute bronchitis and has been subject to treatment and can be discharged on May 25, 2017. His health condition will permit him to return to his work after a week's home rest if the recovery is normal.

(Doctor's Signature)

UNIT SIX

Learning Objectives

After studying this unit, you will be able to:

- ❏ Enlarge your vocabulary related to Lyme disease and the circulatory system;
- ❏ Know how to give a preoperative instruction;
- ❏ Know something about preoperative nursing;
- ❏ Know something about antibiotics and appendicitis;
- ❏ Know something about constipation;
- ❏ Know some prefixes, suffixes or roots of medical terms about the reproductive system;
- ❏ Write a nursing plan and a therapy prescription sheet.

Part 1   Pictures and Charts

Warming-up: Look at the following pictures, talk about them and then finish the task.

Picture 1

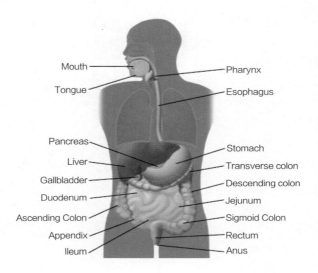

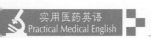
Picture 2

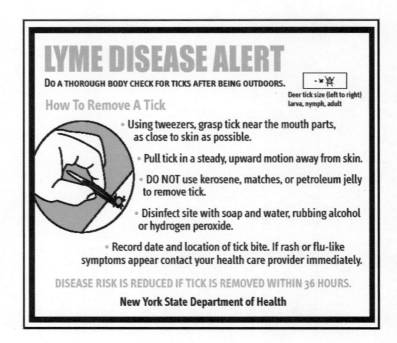

Picture 3

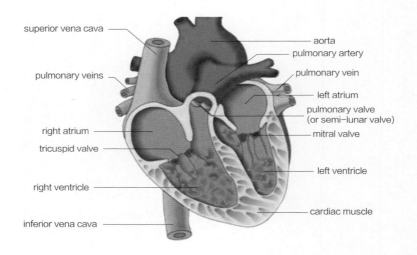

Task: Match the words in the left column with the explanations in the right column.

1.tick	A. a structure in the heart or in a blood vessel that allows blood to flow in one direction only
2.artery	B. any of the tubes forming part of the circulation system by which blood is carried from all parts of the body towards the heart
3.vein	C. each of the two larger and lower cavities of the heart
4.valve	D. a tiny creature related to the spiders, which attaches itself to the skin and sucks blood
5.ventricle	E. any of the tubes through which blood flows from the heart around the body

Part 2   Listening and Speaking

Conversation A

Preoperative Instruction

(A nurse is talking with her patient before an appendectomy.)

Nurse: Good morning, Sir. How are you feeling today?

Patient: I'm not too well. When has Dr. Li, head of the surgery department, decided to perform the appendectomy?

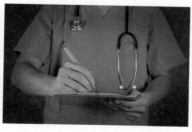

preoperative
/priːˈɒpərətiv/
adj. 外科手术前的
appendectomy
/ˌæpenˈdektəmi/
n. 阑尾切除术

Nurse: I took part in the discussion about your treatment. It was decided that you should undergo surgery the day after tomorrow. I was afraid that you would worry about it, so I've come to put you at ease.

Patient: Yes, I'm very worried.

Nurse: Please don't worry. I'll explain everything to you.

Patient: That's a relief.

Nurse: Now, let me tell you something about what we should do before and after the operation. First of all, you must not eat or drink anything, even water, in preparation for surgery. So, you must keep your stomach empty from 10:00 p.m. tomorrow until the following morning.

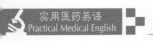
Patient: Ok.

Nurse: Secondly, we must take care that you do not catch a cold or run a fever. The day before the operation, the anesthetists will come to visit you and select the most suitable anesthetics for you. Then, we'll let you have a good night's sleep.

anesthetic /ˌænəsˈθetɪk/ n. 麻醉剂

Patient: I see.

Nurse: Thirdly, we'll take you to the operating theatre and introduce you to the medical staff there.

Patient: Can I eat anything after the operation?

Nurse: No, you will be given intravenous infusions, not only during, but even after the operation. You should stick to a liquid diet for a while, but only eat after breaking wind.

Patient: Thank you. When will I be able to leave the hospital?

Nurse: Commonly, recovery from appendectomy takes a few weeks. Then, you can go home if everything goes smoothly. Before you leave, I will tell you how to take care of yourself at home.

Patient: Thanks. You have really put my mind at ease.

Nurse: You are welcome.

(312 words)

Conversation B

Preoperative Nursing

Task 1: Watch episode one and fill in the missing words referring to the original text. Then check your writing against the original.

Nurse: Morning, Mrs. Peter. I am Cathy. Did you sleep well last night?

Patient: Morning, Cathy. I was a little nervous about the _____, so I didn't sleep that well.

Nurse: Yes, it's hard for everyone at this point. Do you have any questions about the surgery?

Patient: Mm, I signed the consent form two days ago, and I saw the _____ of the operation in the form, such as the complications from the _____, the _____, and even death. I am a little afraid of these things.

Nurse: (*smiles and touches the patient's hand*) I understand it's not easy for you. Actually the consent form tells us all kinds of possibilities during the surgery, but these risks are very small and not likely to happen to you. It's just _____ hospital procedure.

Patient: I see. I hope my surgery is successful. Especially my child is only five years old.

Nurse: (smiles) It will be fine. You should trust the doctors. And you have been on a _____ diet for 3 days, right?

Patient: Yes. May I eat today?

Nurse: Yes, but only clear _____ for today. Then you'll start NPO after midnight.

Task 2: Watch episode two and complete the answers according to the questions.

When will the patient be given an enema?

The patient should be given an enema tonight _____.

Why will the patient be given an enema?

The enema causes the patient to have a _____ and then lower the risk of contamination from the bowel content.

What are two more things before the surgery?

Tomorrow morning the patient will be given a nasogastric tube to keep the _____ empty. And the patient will keep tube for a few days for gastric decompression.

Part 3　Reading Comprehension

Text A

Overuse of Antibiotics

Experts fear antibiotic resistance puts humans in danger of becoming nearly defenseless against some bacterial infections. The World Health Organization calls antibiotic resistance one of the three greatest threats to human health.

resistance /rɪˈzɪstəns/
n. 抵抗力

The improper use of antibiotics has led to strains of bacteria that are resistant to antibiotics. Experts say if efforts to combat the problem are not launched now, infections that were curable could make a dangerous comeback. Dr. Thomas Frieden, director of the U.S. Centers for Disease Control and Prevention, calls on American lawmakers to address the problem.

"If we don't improve our response to the public health problem

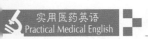

of antibiotic resistance, we may enter a post-antibiotic world in which we will have few or no clinical interventions for some infections," he says.

Specialists are concerned that the more an antibiotic is used, the less effective it becomes. The genetic mutation of bacteria, which makes them resistant to antibiotics, is a natural process. But drug overuse has accelerated the process.

mutation /mju:'teɪʃən/
n. (生物细胞内的) 突变

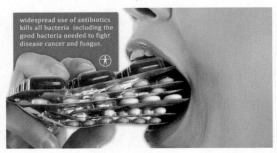

"You end up with very resistant bacteria in the urinary tract. That's only one example. Skin infections, lung infections, different bacteria causing these types of infections as they become more and more resistant, and then you get to a more severe problem like tuberculosis in many parts of the world," says Dr. Donald Poretz, an infectious disease specialist. "People are given little of this and little of that to treat tuberculosis and tuberculosis germs develop resistance."

tuberculosis
/tju:bɜːkjʊ'ləʊsɪs/
n. 结核病
germ /dʒɜːm /
n. 细菌，病菌

"You can have worldwide resistance, different resistance to different drugs in different parts of the world," he says. "And with rapid travel you can communicate those resistant bacteria to anyone here or there."

Experts say the solution lies in educating patients and doctors to stop using antibiotics when they are not necessary.

(291 words)

Text B

Appendicitis

The appendix is a small, tube-like structure attached to the first part of the large intestine, also called the colon. The appendix is

appendicitis
/ə,pendɪ'saɪtɪs/
n. 阑尾炎
appendix /ə'pendiks/
n. 阑尾
colon /'kəʊlən/ n. 结肠

located in the lower right portion of the abdomen, near where the small intestine attaches to the large intestine.

abdomen /ˈæbdəmən/
n. 腹部

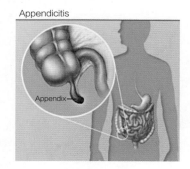

Appendicitis is a condition characterized by inflammation of the appendix. It's most common in the second and third decade of life, but may occur in the very young or old. Males are afflicted in somewhat greater numbers than females.

characterize
/ˈkærɪktəraɪz/
vt. 具有······的特征

The cause of appendicitis relates to blockage of the inside of the appendix, known as the lumen. The blockage leads to increased pressure, impaired blood flow, and inflammation. If the blockage is not treated, gangrene and rupture (breaking or tearing) of the appendix can result.

blockage /ˈblɒkɪdʒ/
n. 阻塞
lumen /ˈluːmen/ *n.* 内腔

gangrene /ˈgæŋɡriːn/
n. 坏疽

Most commonly, feces blocks the inside of the appendix. Also, bacterial or viral infections in the digestive tract can lead to swelling of lymph nodes, which squeeze the appendix and cause obstruction.

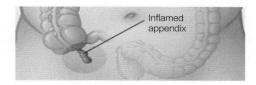

The appendix is a narrow, finger-shaped pouch that projects out from the colon. Appendicitis occurs when the appendix becomes inflamed and filled with pus.

The symptoms of appendicitis are varied. The main symptom of appendicitis is pain that typically begins around your navel and then shifts to your lower right abdomen. The pain of appendicitis usually increases over a period of 6 to 12 hours, and eventually may become very severe. Nausea and vomiting may develop some time after the onset of the pain. Fever is usually present but is seldom

navel /ˈneɪvəl/ *n.* 肚脐

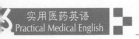

high in the early phase of the disease. Tenderness develops in the right lower abdomen, and the sudden release of pressure of the palpating hand may cause pain.

Because the symptoms of appendicitis can be so similar to those of other medical conditions, it is often a challenge for doctors to diagnose it. When there is some variation in the anatomical location of the appendix the pain and tenderness may be misleading. If the appendix is lateral to or behind the cecum, the tenderness may be in the right flank. If the appendix lies deep in the pelvis one may detect tenderness only on rectal or pelvic examination and even then it may not be easily demonstrated. When the appendix lies on the left side due to the transposition of viscera or failure of normal bowel rotation during embryonic life, the symptoms occur on the left.

tenderness /'tendənɪs/
n. 柔和

palpate /'pælpeɪt/
vt. 触诊

lateral /'lætərəl/
adj. 横（向）的，侧面的
cecum /'si:kəm/ *n.* 盲肠
flank /flæŋk/
n. 腰窝，肋腹
pelvis /'pelvɪs/ *n.* 骨盆
rectal /'rektəl/ *adj.* 直肠的
embryonic /ˌembrɪ'ɒnɪk/
adj. 胚胎的

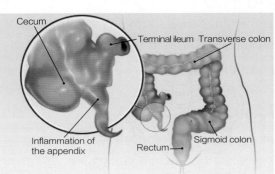

Surgery to remove the appendix, which is called an appendectomy, is the standard treatment for appendicitis. Antibiotics are given before an appendectomy to fight possible peritonitis. General anesthesia is usually given, and the appendix is removed through a 4-inch incision or by laparoscopy. If you have peritonitis, the abdomen is also irrigated and drained of pus.

Generally recovery from appendectomy takes a few weeks. Doctors usually prescribe pain medication and ask patients to limit physical activity. Recovery from laparoscopic appendectomy is generally faster, but limiting strenuous activity may still be necessary for 4 to 6 weeks after surgery. Most people treated for appendicitis recover excellently.

peritonitis /ˌperɪtə'naɪtɪs/
n. 腹膜炎
anesthesia /ˌænɪs'θi:zɪə/
n. 麻醉（anasthesia 的美式拼法）
incision /ɪn'sɪʒən/
n.（手术的）切痕，切口
laparoscopy
/ˌlæpə'rɒskəpɪ/
n. 腹腔镜检查
irrigate /'ɪrɪgeɪt/
vt. 冲洗（伤口）
pus /pʌs/ *n.* 脓，脓汁
strenuous /'strenjʊəs/
adj. 剧烈的

(478 words)

Text C

Constipation

Constipation is a common digestive system problem in which you have infrequent bowel movements, pass hard stools, or strain during bowel movements. There may not be defecation for more than a few days.

Not having a bowel movement every day doesn't necessarily mean you're constipated. You're likely constipated, however, if you:

- pass a hard stool fewer than three times a week;
- strain frequently during bowel movements;
- have abdominal bloating or discomfort.

To understand constipation, it helps to know how the colon, or large intestine, works. As food moves through the colon, the colon absorbs water from the food while it forms waste products, or stool. Muscle contractions in the colon then push the stool toward the rectum. By the time stool reaches the rectum it is solid, because most of the water has been absorbed.

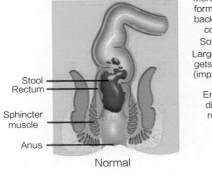

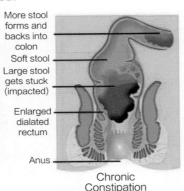

Stool
Rectum

Sphincter muscle

Anus

Normal

More stool forms and backs into colon

Soft stool

Large stool gets stuck (impacted)

Enlarged dialated rectum

Anus

Chronic Constipation

Constipation occurs when the colon absorbs too much water or if the colon muscle contractions are slow or sluggish, causing the stool to move through the colon too slowly. As a result, stools can become hard and dry. Common causes of constipation are:

- inadequate fluid intake;
- a low-fiber diet;

constipation
/ˌkɒnstɪˈpeɪʃən/
n. 便秘
bowel /ˈbaʊəl/ n. 肠
stool /stuːl/ n. 粪便
defecation /ˌdefəˈkeɪʃən/
n. 排便

contraction /kənˈtrækʃən/
n.（肌肉）挛缩
rectum /ˈrektəm/ n. 直肠

intake /ˈɪnteɪk/ n. 摄入量

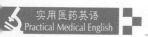

- inattention to bowel habits;
- age;
- lack of physical activity;
- pregnancy;
- illness.

pregnancy /'pregnənsi/
n. 怀孕

When you are constipated you feel that passing stools has become more difficult than it used to be. Passing stools may feel more difficult for one, or more, reasons. For example, passing stools may have become significantly less frequent, or significantly less effective (you feel that you are unable to empty your bowel completely).

significant /sɪg'nɪfɪkənt/
adj. 明显的

Most people do not need to worry extraordinarily. Only a small number of patients with constipation have a more serious medical problem. If you have constipation for more than two weeks, you should see a doctor so he or she can determine the source of your problem and treat

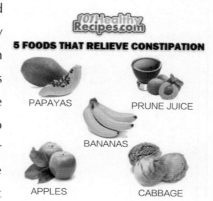

5 FOODS THAT RELIEVE CONSTIPATION

PAPAYAS   PRUNE JUICE
BANANAS
APPLES   CABBAGE

it. If constipation is caused by colon cancer, early detection and treatment are very important.

Diagnosis of constipation generally depends on your medical history and physical exam. Your doctor will first want to make sure you don't have a blockage in your small intestine or colon (intestinal obstruction), an endocrine condition, such as hypothyroidism, or an electrolyte disturbance. He or she will also want to check your medications in case they may be causing your constipation.

intestinal /ˌintes'taɪnl/
adj. 肠的
hypothyroidism
/haɪpəʊ'θaɪrɔɪdɪzəm/
n. 甲状腺机能减退
electrolyte /ɪ'lektrəlaɪt/
n. 电解质
consume /kən'sju:m/
vt. 吃
linseed /'lɪnsi:d/
n. 亚麻子，亚麻仁
laxative /'læksətɪv/
n. 通便剂

For people without medical problems, the main intervention is to increase the intake of fluids (preferably water) and dietary fiber. The latter may be achieved by consuming more vegetables and fruit and wholemeal bread, and by adding linseeds to one's diet. The routine non-medical use of laxatives

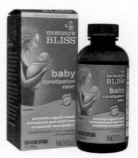

is to be discouraged as this may result in bowel action becoming dependent upon their use. Enemas can be used to provide a form of mechanical stimulation. However, enemas are generally useful only for stool in the rectum, not in the intestinal tract.

stimulation /ˌstɪmjuˈleɪʃən/ n. 刺激

(476 words)

Exercises

Task 1   Oral Practice

Direction: Try to make a conversation about receiving a patient with appendicitis. You can use the following expressions for reference.

I have got pains in my abdomen.

When did the pain start?

Can you tell me the character of the pain?

The pain begins around my navel and then shifts to my lower right abdomen.

Have you ever had this kind of abdominal pain before?

When can I meet the doctor?

The doctor is doing her ward rounds.

The doctor is coming to see you soon.

Doctor, what disease have I got?

I think you have got acute appendicitis.

You should be admitted to an appendectomy.

Do you have any pain in the place where I press?

I'm worried about the operation very much.

Ring any time you need help.

Task 2   Vocabulary Exercise

Direction: Choose the best answers to complete the sentences.

1. _____ is a condition characterized by inflammation of the appendix.

    A. Appendicitis   B. Appendectomy

    C. Appendix   D. Peritonitis

2. The causes of constipation do not include_____.

    A. inadequate fluid intake   B. a low-fiber diet

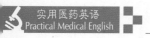

C. inattention to bowel habits   D. quantity of diet

3. By the time stool reaches the_____ it is solid.

    A. intestinal   B. rectum

    C. colon   D. bowel

4. Constipation occurs when the _____ absorbs too much water.

    A. bowel   B. rectum

    C. colon   D. intestinal

5. The cause of appendicitis relates to _____ of the inside of the appendix.

    A. blockage   B. gangrene

    C. rupture   D. inflammation

6. Surgery to remove the appendix is called a(an)_____.

    A. enema   B. peritonitis

    C. appendectomy   D. anesthesia

7. The symptoms of constipation do not include_____.

    A. passing a hard stool fewer than three times a week

    B. straining frequently during bowel movements

    C. having abdominal bloating or discomfort

    D. pregnancy

8. _____is(are) given before an appendectomy to fight possible peritonitis.

    A. Irrigate   B. Antibiotics

    C. Anesthesia   D. enema

9. In people without medical problems on constipation, the main intervention is to increase the _____of fluids (preferably water) and dietary fiber.

    A. intake   B. intestinal

    C. inflammation   D. incision

10. If the appendix is lateral to or behind the_____, the tenderness may be in the right flank.

    A. navel   B. pelvis

    C. lumen   D. cecum

Task 3   Reading Comprehension

Direction: Answer the following questions according to Text A and Text B.

1. What is the cause of appendicitis?

2. How can a doctor treat constipation?

3. What should the patient do after an appendectomy?

4. What are the causes of constipation?

Task 4   Translation

Direction: Put the passage into Chinese with the help of your dictionary.

Sometimes constipation can lead to complications. These complications include hemorrhoids, caused by straining to have a bowel movement, or anal fissures—tears in the skin around the anus—caused when hard stool stretches the sphincter muscle. As a result, rectal bleeding may occur, appearing as bright red streaks on the surface of the stool. Treatment for hemorrhoids may include warm tub baths, ice packs, and application of a special cream to the affected area. Treatment for anal fissures may include stretching the sphincter muscle or surgically removing the tissue or skin in the affected area.

Task 5   Prefixes, Suffixes and Roots

Direction: Learn the prefixes, suffixes or roots in the table and then choose the best answers.

Reproductive System (生殖系统)

汉语 / 英语	常用词根	例　词
生殖 reproduction	genit(o)-	genital 生殖的；urogenital 泌尿生殖的
子宫 womb	uter(o)- hyster(o)- metr(o)-	uterine 子宫的；extrauterine 子宫外的 hysterotomy 子宫切开术 perimetrium 子宫外膜
膀胱 bladder	vesic(o)- cyst(o)-	vesical 膀胱的；rectovesical 直肠膀胱的 cystitis 膀胱炎；cystostomy 膀胱造瘘术
阴道 vagina	vahin(o)- colp(o)-	vaginitis 阴道炎 colposcopy 阴道镜检查；colpoperineoplasty 阴道会阴成形术
月经 menstruation	men(o)-	menopause 绝经；amenorrhea 闭经
胚胎 embryo	embry(o)-	embryology 胚胎学；tubalembryo 胚胎输卵管

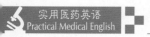

(Continued)

汉语 / 英语	常用词根	例　词
羊膜，羊水 amnion	amni(o)-	amniotic 羊膜的；amniocentesis 羊膜穿刺术； amnioscopy 羊膜镜检查
胎盘 placenta	placent(o)-	placental 胎盘的；uteroplacental 子宫胎盘的
胎儿 fetus	fet(o)-	fetal 胎儿的；fetocardiogram 胎儿心动图
产次 parity	-para	primipara 初产妇；multipara 多产妇
卵泡 follicle	follicul(o)-	follicular 卵泡的；folliculosis 卵泡增殖
卵巢 ovary	ovari(o)-	ovariotomy 卵巢切除术；ovariotubal 卵巢输卵管的
精子 semen	semin(o)-	seminal 精液的；insemination 受精
阴囊 scrotum	scrot(o)-	scrotitis 阴囊炎；scrotectomy 阴囊切除术
阴茎 penis	peni- phall(o)-	penitis 阴茎炎 phallalgia 阴茎痛

1. The Chinese meaning for the word "genital" is _____
   A. 生殖   B. 泌尿生殖的
   C. 生殖的   D. 生殖器

2. The correct medical term for " 阴道炎 " is _____
   A. vulvitis   B. vulvovaginitis
   C. vulvaginiti   D. vaginitis

3. " 子宫切开术 " is called as _____
   A. hysterotomy   B. uterotomy
   C. metrotomy   D. wombotomy

4. The correct interpretation of the word "amenorrhea" is _____
   A. 月经   B. 绝经
   C. 闭经   D. 月经不调

5. The correct spelling for the word " 羊膜 " is _____
   A. amino   B. amnion
   C. ammino   D. annion

6. Fill in the blank with the combining part for the medical term " 羊膜穿刺术 ":
   _____-centesis.
   A. amnio   B. amnion

C. ammio
D. annio

7. The correct interpretation of the word "scrotitis" is _____.

   A. 阴茎痛
   B. 阴茎炎

   C. 阴囊炎
   D. 阴囊肿大

8. The correct Chinese equivalent for the word "tubalembryo" is _____.

   A. 胚胎学
   B. 胚胎

   C. 输卵管
   D. 胚胎输卵管

9. The woman delivering the baby for the first time is called as _____.

   A. deutiapara
   B. nullipara

   C. primipara
   D. multipara

10. The correct spelling for the word "胎儿心动图" is _____.

   A. fetocardiogram
   B. fetal cardiogram

   C. fetus cardiogram
   D. embryo cardiogram

Task 6 Practical Writing

Direction: Read the following practical writing samples carefully and then design a similar nursing plan of recovery from other operations and a therapy prescription sheet by yourself.

Sample 1

A Nursing Plan of Recovery from Appendectomy

Nursing Diagnosis	Nursing Objective	Nursing Measures
Anxiety: associate with lack of knowledge about appendicitis	The patient's anxiety is alleviated or remitted.	Console the patient. Instruct the patient to acquire the knowledge about appendicitis.
Pain: associate with appendicitis and incision of appendectomy	The patient feels the pain has been eased or remitted.	Make the patient occupy a semi-reclining position. Keep the incision dry. Give anodyne to the patient.
Potential complications: bleeding, infection of the incision	The complications can be discovered duly.	Administer antibiotics to the patient.

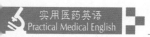
Sample 2

Inhalation Therapy Prescription Sheet

MR 200-3

Flinders Medical Centre

INHALATION THERAPY
PRESCRIPTION SHEET

AFFIX PATIENT LABEL HERE

ALERT [(list drugs) causing/suspected of causing serious adverse event]		WEIGHT	

DATE→ TIME ↓							

DRUG & FORM (Print)		DOSE		0100							
				0200							
				0300							
				0400							
DILUENT (Print)		VOLUME		0500							
				0600							
				0700							
FREQUENCY	Start Time	Start Date		0800							
				0900							
				1000							
M.O. (Sign & Print)				1100							
				1200							
FREQUENCY	Start Time	Start Date		1300							
				1400							
				1500							
M.O. (Sign & Print)				1600							
				1700							
FREQUENCY	Start Time	Start Date		1800							
				1900							
				2000							
M.O. (Sign & Print)				2100							
				2200							
PHARMACY				2300							
				2400							

DRUG & FORM (Print)		DOSE		0100							
				0200							
				0300							
				0400							
DILUENT (Print)		VOLUME		0500							
				0600							
				0700							
FREQUENCY	Start Time	Start Date		0800							
				0900							
				1000							
M.O. (Sign & Print)				1100							
				1200							
FREQUENCY	Start Time	Start Date		1300							
				1400							
				1500							
M.O. (Sign & Print)				1600							
				1700							
FREQUENCY	Start Time	Start Date		1800							
				1900							
				2000							
M.O. (Sign & Print)				2100							
				2200							
PHARMACY				2300							
				2400							

UNIT SEVEN

Learning Objectives

After studying this unit, you will be able to:

- ❑ Enlarge your vocabulary related to the male reproductive system, skeleton and bones;
- ❑ Know how to give a morning shift;
- ❑ Know something about postoperative nursing;
- ❑ Know some common expressions about first aid;
- ❑ Know something about bone fracture;
- ❑ Know some prefixes, suffixes or roots of medical terms about the endocrine system;
- ❑ Write a drug label and a diabetes management flow sheet.

Part 1   Pictures and Charts

Warming-up: Look at the following pictures, talk about them and then finish the task.

Picture 1

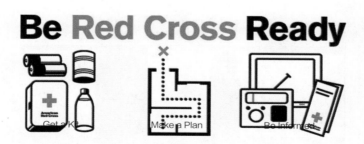

Picture 2

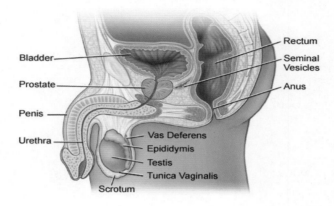

Male Reproductive Tract

Bladder

Prostate

Penis

Urethra

Rectum

Seminal Vesicles

Anus

Vas Deferens

Epididymis

Testis

Tunica Vaginalis

Scrotum

Picture 3

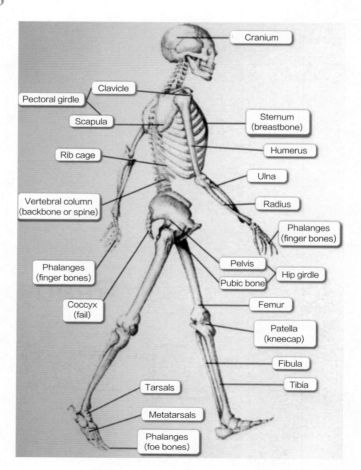

Cranium

Clavicle

Pectoral girdle

Scapula

Sternum (breastbone)

Rib cage

Humerus

Ulna

Vertebral column (backbone or spine)

Radius

Phalanges (finger bones)

Phalanges (finger bones)

Pelvis

Hip girdle

Pubic bone

Coccyx (fail)

Femur

Patella (kneecap)

Fibula

Tibia

Tarsals

Metatarsals

Phalanges (foe bones)

Task: Match the words in the left column with the explanations in the right column.

1. urethra	A. a sac in the abdomen which stores urine for excretion
2. prostate	B. the duct through which urine is conveyed out of the body, and also through which the semen of males flows
3. bladder	C. a gland surrounding the neck of the bladder in male mammals that produces a component of semen
4. pelvis	D. each of a series of thin curved bones attached in pairs to the spine and curving round to protect the chest
5. rib	E. the large bony frame at the base of the spine to which the lower limbs are attached

Part 2   Listening and Speaking

Conversation A

Morning Shift Report

(A nurse in the surgical department is handing over things to the next shift in the office at 8 o'clock in the morning. All of the medical workers in the department are listening.)

shift /ʃift/ n. 轮班

MOTHER-BABY ASSIGNMENTS

M.D. ON DUTY : DR. ALAN R. PETERSON
CHARGE NURSE: SOIBAN KEARNY, N.P.

NURSE	KATHLEEN HAMILTON		NURSE	MICHELLE ROMANA	
RM	PATIENT		RM	PATIENT	
210	DEBORAH JULLIEN●●	LACTATION CONSULT REQUESTED	224	NANCY BARBOUR ●●	
208	BRIDGET O'REILLY●●		221	COLLEEN ROSE	
213	SUSAN ZAJKOWSKI●	BABY SENT TO NICU	220	ALYSSA DEFRANK●	SUSPECT P.P.D.
211	YOLANDA VARGAS ●		222	LORI STANFORD●	
			225	JANET WALSH ●●●	

NURSE	DIANA TUTESBURY		NURSE	VALERIE WILLIAMS	
RM	PATIENT		RM	PATIENT	
215	LISA TIBALDI ●		229	ANN ZIMECKIS ●●	LAC
214	KRISTEN BURDICK●●	MONITOR BLOOD GLUC. LEVEL	226	TERESA MARCONE ●	
219	JILL GOLDSMITH ●●	TREATING FOR STREP.	228	DENISE HALTER ●●	
217	MOLLY SHEILDS ●		230	FAITH MCGANNON ●	
	SABRINA LEWIS ●●●	BABY SENT TO NICU			

Nurse: The total number of patients in our department is 46. On my shift, 2 patients were discharged, 3 patients were newly admitted, and unfortunately 1 patient died.

Head Nurse: Which patients were discharged?

discharge /dɪs'tʃɑːdʒ/ vt. 通知出院
admit /əd'mɪt/ vt. 接纳入院

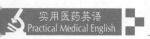
Nurse: Bed No. 3, Li Mei, who suffered from acute appendicitis, recovered after the operation. Bed No.12, Zhang Min, who has breast cancer, left the hospital after her third treatment of chemotherapy.

Head Nurse: How about the deceased patient?

Nurse: Bed No. 8, Wu Ming, male, 50 years old. When he was admitted due to spleen rupture at 4:30 p.m. yesterday, the patient was in a deep coma. Blood pressure: 74/46mmHg; temperature: 36.5℃ ; pulse rate: 98 times/minute. We gave him a blood transfusion and other emergency treatments. However, the treatments were not effective and the patient expired at 5:15 p.m. We have notified his close relatives.

Head Nurse: Well, please tell us something about the 2 new inpatients.

Nurse: Bed No. 12, Wang Li, female, was admitted because she complained of a tumour in the left side of her neck. The etiology is yet to be identified. Another inpatient, Bed No.31, Liu Wei, male, has had intermittent pain in his stomach for the last 2 days. The cause is unclear.

(242 words)

acute /ə'kju:t/
adj. 急性的；严重的
chemotherapy /ˌki:məu'θerəpi/
n. 化学疗法
deceased /dɪ'si:st/
adj. 已故的
spleen /spli:n/ n. 脾脏
coma /'kəumə/ n. 昏迷

expire /ɪk'spaɪə/ vi. 死亡

complain /kəm'pleɪn/ vi. 述说有……病痛

intermittent /ˌɪntə'mɪtənt/ adj. 间歇的

Conversation B

Postoperative Nursing Discussion

Task 1: Watch episode one and fill in the missing words referring to the original text. Then check your writing against the original.

Head Nurse: Hello, everyone. Let's start with Mrs. John. Mrs. John is a 40-year-old American lady and was _____ last Friday. From her biopsy she was diagnosed with rectum cancer 6 months ago in our hospital. A colostomy was performed on her at 10 a.m. yesterday. She is fully awake and _____ from the procedure. We are going to talk about her nursing implementation, especially the stoma care after the surgery.

Nurse 1: Mm, I examined her yesterday after she came back from the OR. I feel that she's doing well. Her _____ signs are good, except for a slight fever. But that's _____ after the surgery. The stoma is swollen, but the _____ _____ around the stoma is good.

Nurse 2: Yes, we need to pay close attention to the stoma.

Head Nurse: What kind of stoma is normal, post-op?

Nurse 1: Stoma is initially edematous and shrinks over next 4 to 6 weeks. A normal stoma is moist and reddish pink. I think Mrs. John's is a standard.

Task 2: Watch episode two and complete the answers according to the questions.

1. What's the first step of the pouching system?

The first step is _____ our hands and apply _____ _____.

2. What should we do after the removal of I the protective backing?

Apply_____ _____.

3. What should do, if the pouch is open?

Don't forget _____ end of the pouch if it is open.

Part 3   Reading Comprehension

Text A

Give Me a Break

The medical term for a broken bone is a fracture. But there are different kinds of fractures.

A single fracture is when a bone is broken in just one place. You may have heard the term hairline fracture. This is a single fracture that is very small, like the width of a hair. A complete fracture is when the bone comes apart. When a bone is broken in more than two places or gets crushed, the name for it is a comminuted fracture. Still another kind is a greenstick fracture. This happens with a bone that bends but does not break, like a young stick of wood. It happens mostly in children. Another kind of break is an open or compound fracture. This is when the bone breaks the skin. This is very serious. Along with the bone damage there is a risk of infection in the open wound.

A lot of things happen as the body reacts to an injury like a

fracture /fræktʃə/ n. 骨折

comminute /kɒmɪnjuːt/ vt. 粉碎

compound /kɒmpaʊnd/ n. 混合体

react /rɪˈækt/ vi. 反应

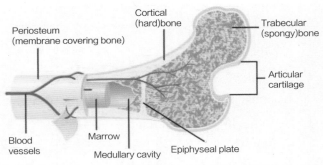

Periosteum (membrane covering bone)

Cortical (hard)bone

Trabecular (spongy)bone

Articular cartilage

Blood vessels

Marrow

Medullary cavity

Epiphyseal plate

broken bone. You might suddenly feel lightheaded. You might also feel sick to your stomach. People who are seriously injured can go into shock. They might feel cold, dizzy and unable to think clearly. Shock requires immediate medical attention. But while broken bones can be painful, they are generally not life-threatening.

shock /ʃɒk/ *n.* 休克

Treatment depends on the kind of fracture. A doctor takes X-rays to see the break and sets a broken bone to make sure it is in the correct position. Severe breaks may require an operation to hold the bone together with metal plates and screws. Next, a person usually gets a cast put around the area of the break. The hard bandage holds the bone in place while it heals. Casts are usually worn for one to two months. In some cases, instead of a cast, a splint made of plastic or metal will be secured over the area to restrict movement. Doctors say broken bones should be treated quickly because they can restrict blood flow or cause nerve damage. Also, the break will start to repair itself, so you want to make sure the bone is lined up correctly.

X-ray /'eks rei/ *n.*
X 光检查

metal plates 金属板
screw /skru:/ *n.* 螺钉
cast /kɑ:st / *n.* 模型
bandage/'bændɪdʒ/
n. 绷带
heal /hi:l/ *vi.* 康复
splint /splɪnt/ *n.* 夹板
restrict /rɪs'trɪkt/ *vt.* 限制

Bones need calcium and vitamin D to grow and reach their full strength. Keeping your bones strong with exercise may also help prevent fractures. Wearing safety protection like elbow pads and leg

calcium /'kælsiəm/ *n.* 钙

Osteoporosis

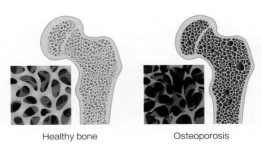

Healthy bone

Osteoporosis

guards during activities is a good idea. If you think these might be restrictive, try a cast.

(403 words)

Text B

First Aid

First aid is the provision of initial emergent care for an illness or injury. It is usually carried out by a lay person to a sick or injured patient until professional medical treatment can be got. Certain illnesses or minor injuries may not require further medical care. It generally consists of a series of simple life-saving techniques that an individual can be trained to perform with minimal equipment.

provision /prə'vɪʒən/
n. 提供
lay /leɪ/ *adj.* 外行的

minimal /'mɪnɪməl/
adj. 极少的

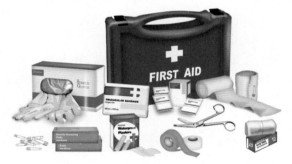

According to the Office for National Statistics in Britain, the top five home accidents and injuries are falls, strikes and collisions, cuts and tears, foreign bodies, acute overexertion, for example moving furniture.

collision /kə'lɪʒən/
n. 碰撞
overexertion
/,əʊvərɪg'zɜːʃən/
n. 努力过度

American College of Emergency Physicians suggests the following ways to prevent medical emergencies.

- Get yearly doctor's exams and regular exercise.
- Protect your health by determining whether you're at risk for any life-threatening conditions, and follow your doctor's suggestions to reduce any risk factors. For example, if you don't smoke, don't start. If you do smoke, quit.
- All medicines should be kept in child-proof containers.
- All poisonous materials should be stored out of reach of children.

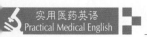

- Drive carefully and appropriately to weather and traffic conditions. All passengers in motor vehicles should wear safety belts.
- Never operate a vehicle if under the influence of alcohol or drugs.
- Read warning labels on all medications to see if they impair your ability to drive or operate machinery.

impair /ɪmˈpeə/
vt. 削弱，损害

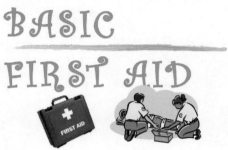

Certain skills are considered essential to the provision of first aid. Particularly, the "ABC" of first aid must be rendered before treatment of less serious injuries. ABC stands for *Airway*, *Breathing*, and *Circulation*. Attention must first be brought to the airway to ensure it is clear. Obstruction (choking) is a life-threatening emergency. Following evaluation of the airway, a first aid attendant would determine the adequacy of breathing and provide oxygen if necessary. Assessment of circulation, typically by checking a carotid pulse determines the need for cardiopulmonary resuscitation.

choke /tʃəuk/ vi. 窒息

carotid /kəˈrɒtɪd/
n. 颈动脉 adj. 颈动脉的
cardiopulmonary
/kɑːdɪəʊˈpʌlmənərɪ/
adj. 心肺的

Some organizations teach the same order of priority using the "3 Bs": *Breathing*, *Bleeding*, and *Bones*. While the ABCs and 3Bs are taught to be performed sequentially, certain conditions may require the consideration of two steps simultaneously. This includes the provision of both artificial respiration and chest compressions to someone who is not breathing and has no pulse.

sequentially /sɪˈkwenʃəlɪ/
adv. 相继地，循序地
simultaneously
/ˌsɪməlˈteɪnɪəslɪ/
adv. 同时地

While some life-saving techniques need training, you can also learn to handle common injuries and wounds. Cuts and scrapes, for example, should be rinsed with cool water. To stop bleeding, apply firm but gentle pressure, using gauze. If blood soaks through, add more gauze, and continue to apply pressure.

scrape /skreɪp/ n. 擦伤
rinse /rɪns/ vt. 冲洗
gauze /ɡɔːz/ n. 纱布

Always remember when to call 120—it is for life-threatening

emergencies in China. It is important to have a first aid kit available. Keep one at home and one in your car. It should include a first-aid guide. Read the guide to learn how to use the items, so you are ready in case an emergency happens.

(487 words)

Text C

Bone Fracture

When external forces are applied to bone it has the potential to fail. Fractures occur when bone cannot withstand those external forces. When a fracture happens, the integrity of the bone has been lost and the bone structure fails.

There are many classifications of fractures according to characteristics such as where they occur and their appearance. A closed fracture means the skin around the fractured bone is not broken. An open one does include a break in the skin, revealing the bone and making the wound more susceptible to infection. A fracture is called complete if the break is the whole way through the bone, and incomplete (or greenstick) if the break is partial. Greenstick fractures are more commonly seen in children. Stress fractures are small cracks in a bone that occur over time as a result of repeated activities that put stress on the bone. According to the way the fracture line goes across the bone, we have a transverse fracture, oblique fracture or spiral fracture. If the fracture is in multiple pieces, it is a comminuted fracture. Actually, a person can have just one fracture or multiple fractures at the same time.

partial /ˈpɑːʃəl/
adj. 局部的

crack /kræk/ *n.* 裂缝

transverse /trænzˈvɜːs/
adj. 横向的
oblique /əˈbliːk/
adj. 倾斜的
spiral /ˈspaiərəl/
adj. 螺旋形的
multiple /ˈmʌltɪpl/
adj. 多重的

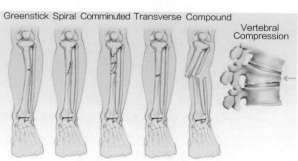

Typical Bone Fractures

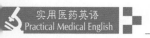

Generally speaking, a bone fracture results in pain, swelling, and sometimes, bruising from internal bleeding. The patient cannot bear weight or pressure on the injured area, and may be unable to move it without severe pain. The soft tissues around the broken bone may also be injured. The area around or below the fracture may feel numb or paralyzed due to a loss of pulse in that area.

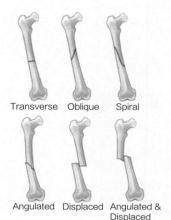

Transverse   Oblique   Spiral

Angulated   Displaced   Angulated & Displaced

bruising /bruːzɪŋ/ n. 瘀青

paralyze /ˈpærəlaɪz/ vt. 使瘫痪，使麻痹

A bone fracture is diagnosed by a physical examination and X-rays of the injured area. However, some types of fractures are difficult to see on an X-ray. In this case, your doctor may order other diagnostic imaging tests, such as computed tomography, magnetic resonance imaging, or bone scans. Open fractures require additional laboratory tests to determine whether blood has been lost and if there is infection.

tomography /təˈmɒɡrəfi/ n. X 线断层摄影术
magnetic /mæɡˈnetɪk/ adj. 有磁性的
resonance /ˈrezənəns/ n. 共振

Initial treatment for fractures of the arms, legs, hands and feet in the field include splinting the extremity in the position it is found, elevation and ice. Immobilization will be very helpful with initial pain control. For injuries of the neck and back, first responders or paramedics may choose to place the injured person on a long board and in a neck collar to protect the spinal cord from potential injury.

immobilization /ɪˌməubəlaɪˈzeɪʃən/ n. 固定

Surgery on fractures is very much dependent on what bone is broken and where it is broken. The bones are manipulated by surgeons so that alignment is restored and a cast is placed to hold the bones in that alignment. Sometimes, the bones are broken in such a way that they need to have metal hardware inserted to hold them in place. Depending on the fracture, some of these pieces of metal are permanent, and some are temporary until the healing of the bone is complete and surgically removed at a later time.

surgery /ˈsɜːdʒəri/ n. 外科手术
manipulate /məˈnɪpjuleɪt/ vt.(熟练地) 操作
alignment /əˈlaɪnmənt/ n. 平行的排列

permanent /ˈpɜːmənənt/ adj. 永久的

(494 words)

Exercises

Task 1   Oral Practice

Direction: Your classroom is a simulation of a general hospital: the classroom front door is the hospital's gate, different groups are different departments in the hospital and the teacher's desk is the hospital information desk. Introduce the hospital to your partner with the following sketch map. You can start your introduction by opening the front door and saying "Welcome to the hospital…"

Isolation Room	Daytime Ward	Medical Lab	Operation Room
Observation Room	Injection Room	X-ray Department	ICU
First Aid Center	Consultation Room	CT room	Inpatient Department
Ambulance	Outpatient Department	Supply Room	EEG Room
Emergency Department	Registration Office	Pharmacy	ECG Room
→ Gate	Information Desk		

Task 2   Vocabulary Exercise

Direction: Match the words or phrases with similar meaning in the two columns.

A	B
1. initial	a. everlasting
2. poisonous	b. nursing staff
3. pulmonary	c. operation
4. fracture	d. man-made
5. immobilization	e. first, beginning
6. permanent	f. toxic
7. paramedic	g. of the lung(s)
8. surgery	h. continuous
9. artificial	i. break
10. sequential	j. fixation

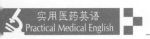

Task 3　Reading Comprehension

Direction: Decide whether the following statements are true or false according to Text A and Text B.

1. The ABCs and 3Bs for first aid are taught to be performed simultaneously.
2. According to the Office for National Statistics, the top five home accidents and injuries in Britain include poisoning.
3. Open fractures require additional laboratory tests to determine whether blood has been lost and if there is infection.
4. For injuries of the neck and back, first responders or paramedics should be careful to protect the spinal cord from potential injury.
5. If the fracture is in multiple pieces, it is an oblique fracture.

Task 4　Translation

Direction: Put the passage into Chinese with the help of your dictionary.

　　How can we prepare for first aid? Keep a list of emergency numbers by the phone. The police, fire department, first aid center, hospital, ambulance service and your family doctor's office should be included. Keep a list of all the medications you and your family take and their dosages. In an emergency, you might not be able to speak for yourself, so carry it with you. The list could help prevent serious drug interactions. Make a list of allergies, particularly drug allergies or those with severe reactions. Keep a well-stocked first-aid kit at home, at work and in your car. A good first-aid kit helps you handle everything from blisters to severe cuts. Take a first-aid class. A basic class will teach cardiopulmonary resuscitation (CPR), and proper methods for treating burns, wrapping sprains, applying splints and performing the Heimlich maneuver.

Task 5　Prefixes, Suffixes and Roots

Direction: Learn the prefixes, suffixes or roots in the table and then choose the best answers.

Endocrine System (内分泌系统)

汉语 / 英语	常用词根	例　词
分泌 secretion	crin(o)- secret(o)-	endocrine 内分泌 secretive 分泌的

汉语 / 英语	常用词根	例　词
腺 gland	aden(o)-	adenoma 腺瘤；adenomyosis 子宫腺肌病
垂体 pituitary	pitui- hypophys-	pituitary 垂体；pituicyte 垂体细胞 hypophyseal 垂体的；hypopituitarism 垂体功能减退
甲状腺 thyroid	thyr(o)-	thyroiditis 甲状腺炎；thyroxine 甲状腺素；thyrotrophin 促甲状腺激素
肾上腺 adrenal	adren(o)-	adrenalitis 肾上腺炎；adrenaline 肾上腺素
胸腺 thymus	thym(o)-	thymosin 胸腺素；thymoma 胸腺瘤
葡萄糖 glucose	gluc(o)-	glucagon 胰高血糖素；glucokinase 葡萄糖激酶
钙 calcium	calc(i)-	calcification 钙化；cholecalciferol 胆钙化醇

1. The correct spelling for the word " 内分泌 " is _____.

    A. endocrine   B. intracrine

    C. intercrine   D. introcrine

2. Fill in the blank with the combining part for the medical term " 子宫腺肌病 ":
_____-myosis.

    A. crino   B. gland

    C. adeno   D. utero

3. The Chinese explanation for the word "hypopituitarism" is _____.

    A. 下丘脑促垂体   B. 垂体功能亢进

    C. 下丘脑垂体   D. 垂体功能减退

4. The Chinese meaning for the word "adenoma" is _____.

    A. 腺瘤   B. 腺癌

    C. 腺素   D. 肾上腺素

5. The correct Chinese equivalent to the word "thymosin" is _____.

    A. 胸腺瘤   B. 胸腺素

    C. 胸腺生成素   D. 胸腺生成

6. Which version of Chinese is right for the term "adrenaline"?

    A. 去甲肾上腺素   B. 肾上腺皮质激素

    C. 肾上腺素   D. 类肾上腺素

7. The English word defined as the inflammation of the thyroid is _____.

    A. thyroiditis   B. adrenalitis

    C. gonaditis   D. thymitis

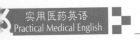

8. The prefix of "calc(i)-" means _____.

    A. kalium

    B. natrium

    C. calcium

    D. iodium

9. The definition of "thymoma" is _____.

    A. any disease of the thymus

    B. tumour of thymus

    C. enlargement of the thymus

    D. hypertrophy of thymus

10. Which term is equal to the English term "cholecalciferol"?

    A. 钙化

    B. 高钙

    C. 降钙素

    D. 胆钙化醇

Task 6　Practical Writing

Direction: Read the following practical writing samples carefully and then write a similar drug direction and a flow sheet for diabetes management.

Sample 1

Drug Directions: Granules for Children's Cold

[Drug Name] Granules for Children's Cold

[Classification] OTC (Over The Counter)

[Description] Light brown granules with a sweet taste

[Compostion] Cablin pacholi, chrysanthemum flower, isatis leaf, isatis root, rehmannia root, wolfberry bark, swallowwort root, peppermint. The auxiliary ingredient is cane sugar.

[Functions and Indications] To dispel wind, clear away heat and eliminate toxic materials. To treat children's wind-heat cold, high fever, headache, cough, sore throat.

[Administration and Dosage] Take the drug with boiled water, two times a day. 6g a time for children under one year, 6 to 12g a time for children from one to three years old, 12 to 18g a time for children from four to seven years old, 24g a time for children from eight to twelve years old.

[Precautions]

1. Cold, uncooked or greasy food is forbidden while taking the medicine.

2. The patients who have watery and frequent stools should not use the medicine.

3. Do not exceed a total of 48g in a day.

[Specification] 12g for each bag

[Storage] Preserve in a tightly closed and moisture-proof container.

[Expiry Date] 2 years from the date of manufacture

Sample 2

Diabetes Management Flow Sheet

DIABETES: TYPE 1 _____ TYPE 2 _____
SBGM: YES _____ NO _____   FREQUENCY: _____
TARGETS: HbA1c _____ SBGM RANGE: PRE-MEAL _____ POST-MEAL _____

DATE(M/D/Y)												
SDM STAGE/PHASE*												
EACH VISIT–REVIEW												
FOOD PLAN												
EXERCISE												
COMPLIANCE**												
MEDICATIONS												
SBGM***												
COMPLICATIONS												
Hypoglycemia												
Chest pain												
Neuropathy												
Claudication												
Vision												
FOOT EXAM (Inspection)												
HbA1c												
Meter Correlation												
ANNUALLY												
COMPLETE FOOT EXAM												
Inspection												
Sensation (Monofilament)												
Pulses												
LIPID												
Total Cholesterol												
HDL												
LDL												
Triglycerides												
PROTEINURIA												
MICROALBUMIN												
DILATED EYE EXAM												

*PHASE–ADJUST OR MAINTENANCE
*STAGES   I –FOOD PLAN/EXERCISE+ORAL MEDICATION
               II –FOOD PLAN/EXERCISE+1–2 DAILY INJECTIONS
               III –FOOD PLAN/EXERCISE+3 DAILY INJECTIONS
               IV –FOOD PLAN/EXERCISE+4 DAILY INJECTIONS
**COMPLIANCE   1=EXCELLENT
                       2=FAIR
                       3=POOR

***–% within target in last 2 wks

UNIT EIGHT

Learning Objectives

After studying this unit, you will be able to:

- ❑ Enlarge your vocabulary related to hospital departments and drug labels;
- ❑ Know how to give health instructions in English;
- ❑ Know something about enema;
- ❑ Know some common expressions about hospital introduction;
- ❑ Know something about leukemia and AIDS;
- ❑ Know some prefixes, suffixes or roots of medical terms about nervous system;
- ❑ Write a nursing flow sheet.

Part 1　Pictures and Charts

Warming-up: Look at the following pictures, talk about them and then finish the task.

Picture 1

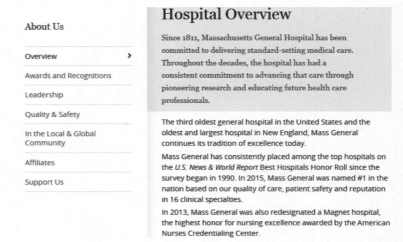

About Us

Overview　　　　　　>

Awards and Recognitions

Leadership

Quality & Safety

In the Local & Global Community

Affiliates

Support Us

Hospital Overview

Since 1811, Massachusetts General Hospital has been committed to delivering standard-setting medical care. Throughout the decades, the hospital has had a consistent commitment to advancing that care through pioneering research and educating future health care professionals.

The third oldest general hospital in the United States and the oldest and largest hospital in New England, Mass General continues its tradition of excellence today.

Mass General has consistently placed among the top hospitals on the *U.S. News & World Report* Best Hospitals Honor Roll since the survey began in 1990. In 2015, Mass General was named #1 in the nation based on our quality of care, patient safety and reputation in 16 clinical specialties.

In 2013, Mass General was also redesignated a Magnet hospital, the highest honor for nursing excellence awarded by the American Nurses Credentialing Center.

Picture 2

Conditions & Treatments	Centers & Departments	Education & Training	Research	Find a Doctor
				Find a Researcher
				Appointments & Referrals

Browse by Medical Category

Allergy & Immunology	Dermatology	Mouth, Teeth & Face
Blood (hematology)	Digestive	Obstetrics & Gynecology
Bones, Muscles and joints (orthopaedics)	Endocrine, Diabetes & Metabolism	Pediatrics
Brain, Spine and Nervous System (neurology & neurosurgery)	Heart	Psychiatry
	Infectious Disease	Rheumatology
Cancer (oncology)	Kidneys	Urology
Circulatory (vascular)	Lung	All Conditions A-Z

FIND CLINICAL TRIALS

Cancer Related Trials   Non-cancer Related Trials

Picture 3

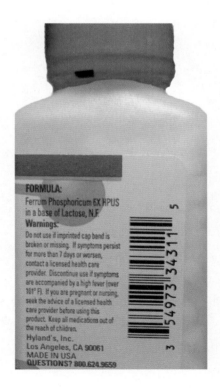

FORMULA:
Ferrum Phosphoricum 6X HPUS
in a base of Lactose, N.F.
Warnings:
Do not use if imprinted cap band is broken or missing. If symptoms persist for more than 7 days or worsen, contact a licensed health care provider. Discontinue use if symptoms are accompanied by a high fever (over 101° F). If you are pregnant or nursing, seek the advice of a licensed health care provider before using this product. Keep all medications out of the reach of children.
Hyland's, Inc.
Los Angeles, CA 90061
MADE IN USA
QUESTIONS? 800.624.9659

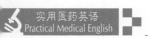

Task: Match the words in the left column with the explanations in the right column.

1. dermatology	A. the branch of medicine concerned with children and their diseases
2. pediatrics	B. a list of ingredients with which something is made
3. psychiatry	C. the branch of medicine concerned with mental illness
4. formula	D. a statement or event that indicates danger or a problem that may or is about to happen
5. warning	E. the branch of medicine concerned with skin disorders

Part 2   Listening and Speaking

Conversation A

Health Instruction

(Mark, an expert from the Centers for Disease Control and Prevention, is giving health instruction about AIDS to Emma, an audience member in the AIDS Prevention Lecture.)

Mark: Hello, everyone. Today we will discuss AIDS. If you have any questions, please don't hesitate to ask me.

Emma: Well, I want to know what AIDS is.

Mark: AIDS stands for "Acquired Immune Deficiency Syndrome", and was first identified in 1981. The virus causing AIDS (called Human Immunodeficiency Virus or HIV) was found in 1983 and a test was developed to detect it in 1985.

acquired /əˈkwaɪəd/ *adj.* 获得的，后天的
deficiency /dɪˈfɪʃənsɪ/ *n.* 不足
immunodeficiency /ˌɪmjuːnəʊdɪˈfɪʃənsɪ/ *n.* 免疫缺陷

Emma: What's HIV?

Mark: Briefly, HIV is a virus. Viruses infect the cells that make up the human body and replicate (make new copies of themselves) within those cells. A virus can also damage human cells, which is one of the things that can make a person ill.

Emma: I also want to know what the most common symptoms of primary HIV infection are.

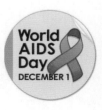

Mark: Fever, aching muscles and joints, sore throat, and swollen glands (lymph nodes) in the neck.

swollen /ˈswəʊlən/ *adj.* 肿胀的
lymph /lɪmf/ *n.* 淋巴
node /nəʊd/ *n.* 节点

Emma: How is HIV passed on?

Mark: There are various ways a person can become infected with HIV, such as: unprotected sexual intercourse with an infected person; contact with an infected person's blood; from mother to child; use of infected blood products, etc.

Emma: How terrible! By the way, is kissing risky?

Mark: Kissing someone on the cheek, also known as social kissing, does not pose any risk of HIV transmission.

Emma: But, how can we prevent AIDS?

Mark: HIV/AIDS prevention is not only a personal action but also a question for the whole society or globe. In the absence of a vaccine to prevent AIDS cases, people control its spread mainly through preventative ways, such as: prevention of sexually transmitted diseases; prevention of blood-borne HIV transmission; prevention of mother-to-child HIV transmission; teaching medical staff to avoid HIV infection.

Emma: Thanks a lot. We have learned so much today.

(323 words)

Conversation B

Enema

Task 1: Watch episode one and fill in the missing words referring to the original text. Then check your writing against the original.

Nurse: Hi, Mrs. John. How are you today ?

Patient: Not bad. How are you?

Nurse: Good. I hear you've been constipated for a few days.

Patient: Yes. I haven't had a bowel movement at least 4 days so my abdomen feels distended and painful. I _____ _____ _____ but it doesn't work.

Nurse: That must be uncomfortable. Dr. Peter _____ an enema for you.

Patient: Oh, what is _____ ? Will it hurt?

Nurse: An enema is a tube of liquid inserted into the rectum through the anus to help your bowel movements. It won't hurt. I am sure you can _____ it.

Patient: Ok, I hope so. What should I do now?

Nurse: You should go to the bathroom first. I'll go to prepare the stuff and come back later.

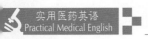

Task 2: Watch episode two and complete the answers according to the question.

1. What does the nurse ask the patient show to her?

The nurse asks the patient to show her _____ bracelet.

2. How should the patient lie?

The patient should take off her pants to the knees and lie _____ _____

_____ _____.

3. How long is the patient asked to keep the position?

The nurse asks the patient to keep the position for _____ _____ _____ minutes.

Part 3　Reading Comprehension

Text A

Florence Nightingale

International Nurses' Day falls on May 12th every year. People celebrate it to commemorate Florence Nightingale, the founder of women vocational nurses, the British nursing pioneer, and the founder of modern nursing education.

commemorate /kə'meməreɪt/ vt. 纪念

May 12th, 1820, Nightingale was born in a wealthy and well-educated family in Florence, Italy. When she was a little girl, she had a merciful and sympathetic heart and nursed the injured animals with kindness and carefulness. She went to Germany studying nursing regardless of objections from her family in 1850.

merciful /'mɜːsɪfəl/ adj. 慈悲的
sympathetic /ˌsɪmpə'θetɪk/ adj. 有同情心的

She went to the Crimean War when the war (1854–1856) broke out there between Britain and Russia. She established the first of what we now know as war-hospital: sanitary, safe, and stocked with supplies. Her tireless care to the wounded soldiers made her famous all over the world. She always carried a light with her in the war-hospital every night, and for this reason she was recognized as Lady with Lamp. In 1857, in her efforts, the British Royal Army Health Committee was established. The same year, the Medical School established.

sanitary /'sænɪtərɪ/ adj. 卫生的

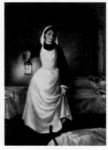

In 1860 she used public funds which were contributed to her established the world's first formal nursing schools—Nightingale Nursing School in St. Thomas Hospital in the U.K. Nightingale has many theoretical works, like Hospital Notebook, Nursing Notes, and other major nursing works, which have been the basic materials in hospital management and nursing education. In 1901, Nightingale was blind which was due to excessive strain. In 1907, the U.K. king issued a merit order to Nightingale, which made her become the first woman to accept the highest honor in history. Nightingale devoted the rest of her life to making public health and standards of hospital care better, taking nursing out of the dark ages and turning it into a skilled and respectable profession. In 1910, Nightingale died at the age of 90. After her death, according to her will, people didn't hold a state funeral for her.

theoretical /ˌθɪəˈretɪkəl/ *adj.* 理论的

excessive /ɪkˈsesɪv/ *adj.* 过度的
strain /streɪn/ *n.* 焦虑

respectable /rɪˈspektəbl/ *adj.* 受人尊敬的
funeral /ˈfjuːnərəl/ *n.* 葬礼

In honor of her major contribution towards nursing career, in 1912, ICN (International Council of Nurses) set her birthday as International Nurses' Day to encourage the majority of nurses in the care to carry on the glorious tradition of Nightingale, keeping on treating every patient with love, patience, care and responsibility. Her birthday has been the centerpiece of National Hospital Week, observed in British and American hospitals with special exhibitions, workshops, and publicity drives.

observe /əbˈzɜːv/ *vt.* 遵守
workshop /ˈwɜːkʃɒp/ *n.* 研讨会，工作坊

(429 words)

Text B

Leukemia

Leukemia is a malignant disease of the hematopoietic system, commonly known as the "cancer of the blood". A large number of uncontrolled proliferation leukemia cells exist in the bone marrow and other hematopoietic tissue, and fluid into the bloodstream and organs to restrain the manufacture of normal blood cells.

There are several types of leukemia. The types of leukemia are mainly distinguished by the types of abnormal blood cells within

leukemia /luːˈkiːmɪə/ *n.* 白血病
malignant /məˈlɪgnənt/ *adj.* 恶性的
hematopoietic /hemətəupɒɪˈiːtɪk/ *adj.* 造血的
marrow /ˈmærəu/ *n.* 骨髓

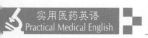
the blood. Leukemia is clinically and pathologically split into its acute and chronic forms. The types of leukemia are also grouped by the type of white blood cell that is affected. Leukemia can arise in lymphoid cells or myeloid cells. Leukemia that affects lymphoid cells is called lymphocytic leukemia. Leukemia that affects myeloid cells is called myeloid leukemia or myelogenous leukemia.

lymphocytic
/ˌlɪmfəˈsaɪtɪk/
adj. 淋巴细胞的
myelogenous
/ˌmaɪəˈlɒdʒənəs/
adj. 骨髓性的

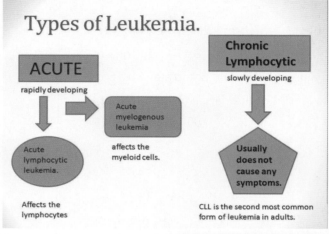

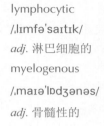

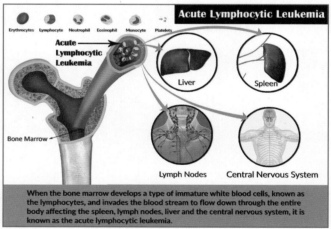

The incidence of leukemia causes has not fully established yet. The study shows it may be related to radiation, some chemicals, virus infections and genetic factors, etc. In the animal and the humanity, the function which irradiation nuclein caused leukemia has been affirmed. A large dose or multiple small doses of radiation can cause leukemia. Benzene has been confirmed as the intense carcinogen by WHO. A long-term inspiration may destroy the human body's circulatory system and the hematopoietic function,

radiation /ˌreɪdɪˈeɪʃ ən/
n. 放射物
nuclein /ˈnjuːklɪɪn/ n. 核素
benzene /ˈbenziːn/ n. 苯
carcinogen /kɑːˈsɪnədʒən/
n. 致癌物
circulatory /sɜːkjʊˈleɪtərɪ/
adj. 血液循环的

which causes leukemia. In recent years, benzene of daily life mainly comes from a lot of chemical industry raw materials used in the construction decoration, such as dope, wood lacquer, adhesive and various organic solvents.

dope /dəʊp/ n. 涂料
lacquer /ˈlækə/ n. 漆
solvent /ˈsɒlvənt/ n. 溶剂

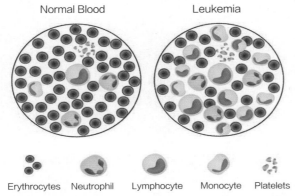

Normal Blood Leukemia

Erythrocytes Neutrophil Lymphocyte Monocyte Platelets

Damage to the bone marrow, by way of displacing the normal bone marrow cells with higher numbers of immature white blood cells, results in the following symptoms:

immature /ˌɪməˈtʃʊə/ adj. 不成熟的

- A lack of blood platelets, which are important in the blood clotting process. This means people with leukemia may become bruised, bleed excessively.

clot /klɒt/ vi. 凝结

- White blood cells may be suppressed or confused excessively, which may affect the patient's immunity.

- The red blood cell deficiency leads to anemia, which may cause dyspnea.

anemia /əˈniːmɪə/ n. 贫血
dyspnea /dɪsˈpniːə/ n. 呼吸困难

Some other related symptoms:

- Mild fever, chills, night sweats and other flu-like symptoms;

- Weakness and fatigue;

- Swollen or bleeding gums;

- Neurological symptoms (headaches);

neurological /ˌnjʊərəˈlɒdʒɪkəl/ adj. 神经学的

- Enlarged liver and spleen;

- Frequent infection;

- Aches in bones or joints (for example, knees, hip or shoulders);

- Dizziness;

- Nausea;

- Swollen lymph nodes, especially in the neck or armpit;

- Diarrhea;

diarrhea /daɪəˈrɪə/ n. 腹泻

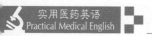

- Paleness;
- Malaise;
- Weight loss.

All symptoms can be attributed to other diseases; for diagnosis, blood tests and a bone marrow examination are required.

attribute /əˈtrɪbjuːt/
vt. 把……归因于

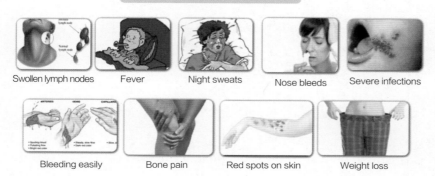

Leukemia Symptoms

Swollen lymph nodes | Fever | Night sweats | Nose bleeds | Severe infections

Bleeding easily | Bone pain | Red spots on skin | Weight loss

Treatment of leukemia depends on the type of leukemia, certain features of the leukemia cells, the extent of the disease, and prior history of treatment, as well as the age and health of the patient. Patients may have chemotherapy, biological therapy, radiation therapy, or bone marrow transplantation. If the patient's spleen is enlarged, the doctor may suggest surgery to remove it. Some patients receive a combination of treatments.

transplantation
/ˌtrænsplɑːnˈteɪʃn/
n. 移植

(495 words)

Text C

AIDS

People have been warned about HIV and AIDS for over twenty years now. AIDS has already killed millions of people and is one of biggest problems facing the world today, and nobody is beyond its reach. Everyone should know the basic facts about AIDS.

AIDS stands for Acquired Immunodeficiency (or Immune Deficiency) Syndrome. It results from infection with a virus called HIV, which stands for Human Immunodeficiency Virus. This disease primarily spread through sexual intercourse and blood. This virus infects key cells in the human body called CD4-positive (CD4+) T cells. These cells are part of the body's immune system, which fights infections and various cancers.

AIDS symptoms of infection have a variety of performance because of the conditions of the internal organs and in different parts of a tumour. Common symptoms in the following areas:

- General symptoms: persistent fever, weakness, night sweats, general superficial lymphadenopathy, weight loss;
- Respiratory symptoms: long-term cough, chest pain, dyspnea, sputum serious blood;
- Gastrointestinal symptoms: such as anorexia, nausea, vomiting, diarrhea, severe blood in the stool;
- Nervous system symptoms: dizziness, headache, unresponsive, decreased intelligence, mental disorders, twitch, hemiplegia and dementia;
- Damage to the skin and mucous membranes: diffuse papule, herpes zoster, inflammation and ulceration on oral and pharyngeal mucosa;
- A variety of malignant tumours, such as Kaposi's sarcoma that represents red or purple macula, papules and invasive tumour.

Therefore, the symptom of AIDS is very complex.

The diagnosis of HIV infection can be made by detecting the presence of disease-fighting proteins called antibodies in the blood. Two different types of antibody tests, enzyme-linked immunoassay (ELISA) and Western blot, are available.

superficial /su:pə'fɪʃəl/ *adj.* 表皮的

lymphadenopathy /ˈlɪmˌfædə'nɒpəθɪ/ *n.* 淋巴结病

anorexia /ˌænə'reksɪə/ *n.* 厌食

hemiplegia /hemɪ'pli:dʒɪə/ *n.* 偏瘫

dementia /dɪ'menʃə/ *n.* 痴呆

herpes /ˈhɜ:pi:z/ *n.* 疱疹 zoster /ˈzɒstə/ *n.* 带，带状疹子

ulceration /ˌʌlsə'reɪʃən/ *n.* 溃疡

macula /ˈmækjʊlə/ *n.* 斑疹

immunoassay /ɪmjʊnəʊ'æseɪ/ *n.* 免疫测定

YOU CAN GET HIV VIA...

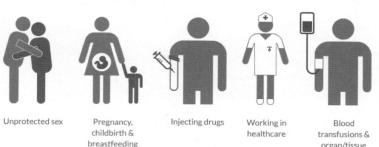

Unprotected sex | Pregnancy, childbirth & breastfeeding | Injecting drugs | Working in healthcare | Blood transfusions & organ/tissue transplants

You can decrease your chances of being infected with HIV by avoiding high-risk behaviors.

- Don't have sex, or have sex with only one partner who is also committed to having sex with only you.
- Use condoms with each act of sexual intercourse.
- If you use intravenous drugs, never share needles.
- If you are a health care worker, strictly follow universal precautions (the established infection-control procedures to avoid contact with bodily fluids).
- If you are a woman thinking about becoming pregnant, have a test for HIV beforehand, especially if you have a history of behaviors that put you at risk of HIV infection. Pregnant women who are HIV-positive need special prenatal care and medications to decrease the risk that HIV will pass to their newborn babies.

condom /'kɒndəm/
n. 避孕套

prenatal /ˌpriː'neɪtl/
adj. 产前的

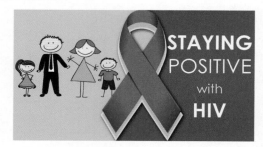

The prevention and treatment for people with HIV have improved enormously since the mid-1990s, but there is still no way to cure AIDS. The general principle of the treatment included anti-infection, anti-tumour, eliminating or restraint the HIV virus and enhancement organism immunity function.

(512 words)

Exercises

Task 1   Oral Practice

Direction: Explain in English the location and function of the following human body organs.

Example:

The tongue is in our mouth and we use it when we speak the language and eat food.

1.tongue	2. stomach	3. eyeball	4. heart	5. brain
6. liver	7. gallbladder	8. pancreas	9. spleen	10. lungs
11.kidney	12. prostate	13.uterus	14. ovary	15. urinary bladder

Task 2   Vocabulary Exercise

Direction: Match the words or phrases with similar meanings in the two columns.

1. immature	a. being on or near the surface
2. anorexia	b. existing or occurring before birth
3. anemia	c. a feeling of sickness or disgust
4. superficial	d. physical or mental weariness resulting from exertion
5. nausea	e. paralysis affecting only one side of the body
6. hemiplegia	f. the condition of the blood caused by a lack of red corpuscles
7. prenatal	g. loss of appetite, esp. as a result of disease
8. macula	h. of or relating to the circulatory system
9. fatigue	i. not fully grown or developed
10. circulatory	j. a spot, stain

Task 3   Reading Comprehension

Direction: Answer the following questions according to Text A and Text B.

1. What are the symptoms of leukemia?
2. What methods can be used to treat leukemia?
3. What is AIDS?
4. What tests can be used to diagnose AIDS?

Task 4   Translation

Direction: Put the passage into Chinese with the help of your dictionary.

People regard AIDS as a terrible disease in the late 1980s. AIDS patients are discriminated against. The Red Ribbon was created in New York in 1991 by the Visual AIDS Artists Caucus—a group of artists who wished to create a visual symbol to demonstrate compassion for people living with HIV/AIDS and their caregivers. Red Ribbon is the symbol of solidarity, care and support of people living with HIV/AIDS; the symbol of our love for life and the desire for peace, the symbol of the determination of the fight against AIDS.

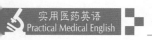

December 1st is the World AIDS Day. Started in 1988, World AIDS Day is not just about raising money, but also about raising awareness, education and fighting prejudice. World AIDS Day is also important in reminding people that HIV has not gone away.

Task 5　Prefixes, Suffixes and Roots

Direction: Learn the prefixes, suffixes or roots in the table and then choose the best answers.

Nervous System (神经系统)

汉语 / 英语	常用词根	例　词
脑 brain	encephal(o)-	encephalitis 脑炎；encephalopathy 脑病；encephalomyelitis 脑脊髓炎
大脑 cerebrum	crecbr(o)-	crecbral 大脑的；crecbrovascular 脑血管的
小脑 cerebellum	cerebell(o)-	archicerebellum 原小脑；cerebrocerebellum 皮层小脑
丘脑 thalamus	thalam(o)-	metathalamus 后丘脑；epithalamus 上丘脑
髓质 marrow	medull(o)-	medullary 髓质的；adrenomedullin 肾上腺髓质素
脑膜，脊膜 membrane	mening(o)-	meningitis 脑膜炎；leptomeningitis 软脑膜炎；pachymeningitis 硬脑膜炎
脊柱 spine	spin(o)-	spinocerebellum 脊柱小脑；cerebrospinal 脑脊的
精神，意志 mind	psych(o)-	psychopathology 精神病理学；psychostimulant 精神兴奋剂
神经 nerve	neur(o)-	neurology 神经病学；neurotmesis 神经断伤
蛛网膜 arachnoid	arachn (o)-	arachnoidal 蛛网膜的；arachnoiditis 蛛网膜炎；subarachnoid 蛛网膜下
狂，癖 madness	-mania(c)	erotomania 色情狂；tocomania 产后躁狂；dipsomania 酒狂

1. The correct spelling of the term "脑血管的" is _____ vascular.

　　A. encephalo-　　　B. brain　　　　　C. cerebro-　　　　D. cerebello-

2. The term "leptomeningitis" can be translated into Chinese term _____.

　　A. 脑膜炎　　　　　B. 软脑膜炎　　　C. 硬脑膜炎　　　　D. 脑膜膨出

3. The correct Chinese meaning of the word "arachnoid" is _____.

　　A. 蛛网膜下　　　　B. 蛛网膜炎　　　C. 蛛网膜下腔　　　D. 蛛网膜

4. The word "subthalamus" means the portion situated _____ the thalamus.

    A. above   B. over   C. under   D. below

5. The branch of medical science that is concerned with nerves is termed as _____.

    A. neurology   B. neuroscience   C. neurobranch   D. nervescience

6. Any degenerative disease of the brain is termed as _____.

    A. encephalitis   B. encephaloma   C. leukoencephalitis D. encephalopathy

7. What does the inflammation in both the brain and the spinal cord mean in medicine?

    A. Encephalomyelitis.   B. Leukoencephalitis.

    C. Encephalitis.   D. Cerebrospinal.

8. The combining part "encephalo-" denotes the relationship to the _____.

    A. brain stem   B. brain   C. large brain   D. small brain

9. The combining part which denotes a relationship to the membranes covering the brain is _____.

    A. encephalo-   B. cerebro-   C. meningo-   D. cerebello-

10. Which combining part denotes the relationship to the madness?

    A.-kinesia   B.-gnosis   C.-phobia   D.-mania

Task 6   Practical Writing

Direction: Read the following practical writing samples carefully and then write a similar e-mail letter and design a nursing flow sheet by yourself.

Sample 1

An E-mail Letter

E-mail Inbox
To: jiaxin@sina.com
From: Helen1127@126.com
Date: Tue., 9 May, 2017,10:18:38
Subject: Thanks a lot
Dear sir,
I am writing this letter to express my deep appreciation to your hospital. Thank you for your warm hospitality and honesty of the staff in your hospital.

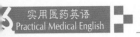

Last week I lost my handbag in your hospital when I visited my friend, a patient who was in hospital. I was very anxious because it was very important to me. It's not an ordinary handbag for it contained $2,000 in cash and a business contact book. I was very disappointed. I didn't believe that someone would return it to me. But I was wrong. The nurse in your hospital found it and handed it to the head nurse office. I was so excited when she phoned me. Thank you for your help!

With kind personal regards!

Yours Sincerely,

Helen

Sample 2

A Nursing Flow Sheet

CONTINUOUS EPIDURAL NURSING FLOW SHEET

Allergies: _____

Procedure: _____ Wt:____kg M:_____ F: _____ Age:_____yrs

CATHTER DEPTH = _____cm EPIDURAL PLACEMENT: Thoracic / Lumbar / Caudal 1 2 3 4 5 6 7 8 9 10

	Data														
	Time														
Pain Score (check scale used)	10														30
☐ NIPS ☐ FLACC	8														24
☐ Modified Faces ☐ Modified CHEOPS	6														18
☐ Comfort Scale	4														12
☐ Numerical Rating Scale	2														6
Drug /Concentration (mg / ml)(mcg / ml)(%)*															
Infusion Rate (ml / hr)															
Bolus Dose (mg)(mcg)															
Syringe Level															
HOURLY INTAKE (ml)															
Total Intake (8 Hours)															
VITAL SIGNS: Blood Pressure															
Temperature															
Heart Rate / Apex															
Respiratory Rate															
Oxygen Saturation (%)															
Sedation Score (S,1–4)															
Bromage Motor Scale															
MD Notified for Scale <4 (√)															
Range of Sensory Dermatome															
(if unequal use R/L)															
Activity **															
Connector / Filter Check (√)															
Dressing/Landmark Check (√)															
Skin Check (√)															
Epidural Caution Labels (√)															
See Nurse's Notes (SNN)															
Nurse's Initials															

ALETRS:

NO SYSTEMIC NARCOTICS, CNS DEPRESSANTS TO BE GIVEN EXCEPT AS ORDERED BY ANESTHESIA
NARCAN (NALOXONE 10 MCG / KG) IMMEDIATELY AVAILABLE & OXYGEN, SELF–INFLATING BAG & SUCTION AVAILABLE AT ALL TIMES
NOTIFY ANESTHESIA IMMEDIATELY IF SEDATION SCORE = 3 OR IF PROGRESSIVE MOTOR BLOCK / RISING SENSORY LEVEL

Key: *Morphine (MO) Fentanyl (FEN) Ropivacaine (ROP) Epinephrine (EPI) Dilaudid (DIL)
**Turning (T), Dangling (D), Chair (C), Walking (W).
Form No. 1055. Rev May 02

UNIT NINE

Learning Objectives

After studying this unit, you will be able to:

- ❑ Enlarge your vocabulary related to supplement facts and WHO;
- ❑ Talk about discharge from hospital;
- ❑ Know how to do health education for diabetic patients;
- ❑ Know something about obesity;
- ❑ Know something about stress;
- ❑ Know some prefixes, suffixes or roots of medical terms about common diseases;
- ❑ Write a nursing record and a medical face sheet.

Part 1 Pictures and Charts

Warming-up: Look at the following pictures, talk about them and then finish the task.

Picture 1

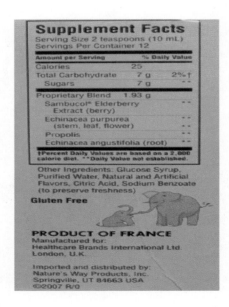

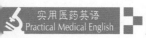

Picture 2

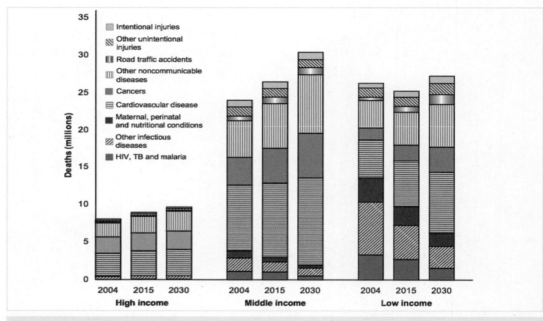

PROJECTED DEATHS BY CAUSE FOR HIGH-, MIDDLE- AND LOW-INCOME COUNTRIES

Picture 3

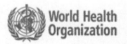

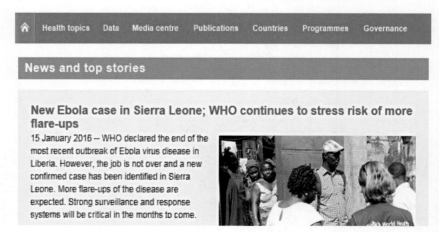

World Health Organization

Health topics   Data   Media centre   Publications   Countries   Programmes   Governance

News and top stories

New Ebola case in Sierra Leone; WHO continues to stress risk of more flare-ups

15 January 2016 — WHO declared the end of the most recent outbreak of Ebola virus disease in Liberia. However, the job is not over and a new confirmed case has been identified in Sierra Leone. More flare-ups of the disease are expected. Strong surveillance and response systems will be critical in the months to come.

Task: Match the words in the left column with the explanations in the right column.

1. calorie	A. any of a large group of compounds (including sugars and starch) which contain carbon, hydrogen, and oxygen, found in food and used to give energy
2. carbohydrate	B. a unit of energy equal to the energy needed to raise the temperature of 1 kilogram of water through 1℃
3. flare	C. suddenly become stronger or violent
4. ingredient	D. a very small living thing that causes infectious diseases
5. virus	E. substance in a product such as a medicine

Part 2   Listening and Speaking

Conversation A

Discharge

(In a ward one morning)

Nurse: Good morning. How are you feeling today?

Patient: I feel much better.

Nurse: I'll take your temperature. Please put the thermometer in your armpit.

armpit /ɑːmͺpɪt/ *n.* 腋窝

(Fifteen minutes later)

Nurse: Please give me the thermometer.

Patient: Thank you.

Nurse: It reads 36.8 degrees centigrade. Do you know you are going to be discharged today?

Patient: That's great. I'm so happy. I have been in hospital for 10 days, but my doctor told me yesterday that I should have one more week of rest.

Nurse: Yes, you need more rest. However, you can go back home to rest, because your general health has improved. The doctor has a discharge certificate for you. I'll get it.

Patient: Thanks a lot. My employer wants my medical records. May I have them?

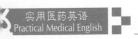
Nurse: Certainly. I'll copy them for you. Your family members can go to the admission office to go through your discharge procedure.

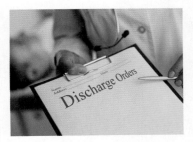

Patient: How much do I owe the hospital? May I pay for it by cheque?

Nurse: Our hospital has given you your daily bill each morning. You can calculate them, or I can do it for you. You can pay for it either by cash or cheque.

Patient: Thank you. Do you have any suggestions for me when I get home?

Nurse: You should try to avoid mental stress, stop smoking, and avoid spicy food.

Patient: Should I do some physical exercises?

Nurse: Of course, it is necessary. Also, you'd better do aerobic exercises. Such exercises as walking, jogging, and Tai Chi are good for the healing process, but you should protect your incision and monitor your blood glucose level after exercising.

aerobic /ˌeəˈrəʊbɪk/
adj. 有氧的

Patient: What can I eat?

Nurse: Anything that is nutritious, but you should stick to a regular diet.

Patient: Thank you, nurse. You have helped a lot.

Nurse: No problem. It is our duty. Keep taking your medicine and come to hospital to have regular examinations. If you feel bad, you should seek professional health care immediately.

(336 words)

Conversation B

Health Education

Task 1: Watch episode one and fill in the missing words referring to the original text. Then check your writing against the original.

Nurse: Hi, Mrs. Peter. How are you today?

Patient: Good. How are you?

Nurse: Very good. Thank you. I'd like to talk about your _____ management before your discharge.

Patient: Oh, thanks. I am really worrying about the complication of the diabetes after I go back home.

Nurse: I understand it's not easy for you to manage it now, so we need to _____ you first.

Patient: I think so.

Nurse: OK, let's start. There are two types of diabetes, type 1 and type 2. Do you know what type you have?

Patient: Type 2. It's also called non-insulin-dependent diabetes. And the doctor suggested me that I take the _____ injections.

Nurse: Good. Can you tell me how many units have been _____ for you?

Patient: 4 units of _____ insulin. But I am not sure.

Task 2: Watch episode two and complete the answers according to the questions.

1. When should the patient inject the insulin?

Remember to inject the insulin 30 minutes _____ _____ _____.

2. Why do most diabetics use insulin pen?

Most diabetics use insulin pen because its prefilled devices are _____ _____ _____for them.

3. According to doctors' orders, what must the patient do in case of hyperglycemia?

The patient must have some _____ according to doctors' orders in case of hyperglycemia.

Part 3   Reading Comprehension

Text A

Childhood Obesity

Since obesity in adolescents has nearly tripled in the past two decades, it is an important topic to discuss. Unfortunately, childhood obesity is a sensitive subject for many and often ignored.

The detrimental effects of obesity on health are multiple,

obesity /əʊ'biːsətɪ/
n. 肥胖
adolescent /ˌædəʊ'lesənt/
n. 青少年
triple /'trɪpl/ vi. 增至三倍
decade /'dekeɪd/ n. 十年
ignore /ɪg'nɔː/ vt. 忽视

associated with an increased risk of heart disease, high blood pressure, type 2 diabetes and various forms of cancer. Metabolic effects have been observed in children as young as 6 years old.

In most cases, an overweight child can lose weight simply by changing his eating habits and lifestyles. Most children spend large amounts of time playing computer games, watching TV, surfing the Internet and spending long hours completing their homework.

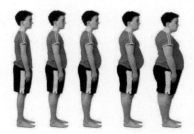

Treating childhood obesity is extremely difficult and the numbers of those who effectively lose weight and maintain this loss are extremely low.

The answer lies in prevention and the key to this is education—teaching kids about obesity and why it happens, what the dangers of obesity are and what "healthy eating" is. It is also crucial to teach children how to cook and avoid dependence on takeaways and fast food, and of course, to highlight the huge importance of exercise.

crucial /ˈkruːʃəl/ *adj.* 极重要的

highlight /ˈhaɪlaɪt/ *vt.* 强调

The Chinese government is certainly aware of the need for action. Once the Chinese Center for Disease Control and Prevention (CDC) released a guide to healthy eating for Chinese children and their parents a direct attempt to slow rising childhood obesity levels.

Former Minister of Education Zhou Ji once stipulated that schools should ensure at least one hour's physical exercise per day.

stipulate /ˈstɪpjəleɪt/ *vt.* 要求

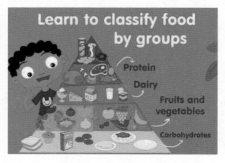

Learn to classify food by groups

Protein

Dairy

Fruits and vegetables

Carbohydrates

Ultimately though, responsibility must lie with the families. Encouraging properly balanced meals at home, along with exercise and discouraging TV and computer games will set a good example to children.

At the National Obesity Forum conference in the UK there was a lively debate as to whether child obesity should be considered a child protection issue based on the premise that the consequences of neglect leading to malnutrition can be just as serious as those leading to obesity. That's certainly something to think about.

(349 words)

forum /ˈfɔːrəm/ *n.* 论坛
premise /premɪs/ *n.* 前提
neglect /nɪˈglekt/ *n.* 疏忽
malnutrition
/ˌmælnjʊˈtrɪʃən/
n. 营养不良

Text B

Obesity

Obesity refers to the condition with too much body fat, which is usually regarded as unhealthy. Medically, it is different from overweight. For weight comes from fat, muscle, bone, and body fluids. Obesity is an out-coming of long-term overtaking fat or calories.

overweight /ˌəʊvəˈweɪt/
n. 超重
calorie /kælərɪ/ *n.* 卡路里

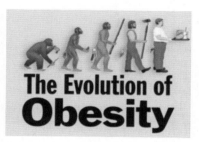

Many ways are used to determine whether a person is overweight or not. But health care professionals believe that the body mass index (BMI) is the most accurate measurement.

Metric: $BMI = kg/m^2$

metric /ˈmetrɪk/
n. 度量标准

Where the *kg* is the individual's weight in kilogram, and the *m* is the height in meter. In 1997, the World Health Organization (WHO) set up the following values:

• A BMI less than 18.5 is *underweight;*

• A BMI of 18.5–24.9 is *normal weight;*

• A BMI of 25.0–29.9 is *overweight;*

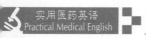

- A BMI of 30.0–39.9 is *obese;*

- A BMI of 40.0 or higher is *severely (or morbidly) obese.*

Calories balance is of great importance to be away from obesity.

Many factors contribute to obesity: energy balance, physical activity, environment, genes, family history, health condition, medicine, emotional factors, age, smoking, pregnancy, and lack of sleep. Energy is balanced by the amount got from food equaling to that used by such activities as working, breathing and digesting. When there is more energy taken in than that used out, the individual is gaining weight. In contrast, the individual is losing weight. Therefore, obesity occurs over a long time when the body takes more energy than that used out.

obese /əʊˈbiːs/
adj. 肥胖的
morbidly /ˈmɔːbɪdlɪ/
adv. 病态地

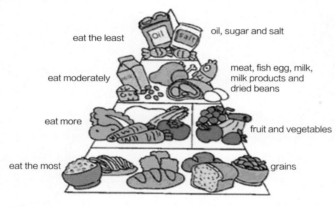

In modern society, there are increasing numbers of people who are physically inactive. Depart from the 8 hours during which people have to sit at their working desk, modern people spend many of their spare-time hours watching TV programs, surfing the Internet or muddling with strangers online. Actually, it is said that more than 2 hours a day of regular TV viewing time has been linked to obesity. Other factors also would reduce the physical activity time. Modern technologies provide more convenience and decrease the need for body activities and lessen calorie burning. More people drive cars rather than walk to the offices.

The environment would change people's lifestyle and food health. The crowded neighborhood provides fewer community parks and sidewalks. A large scale of food portions, high calorie and high-fat food advertisements increase people's probability to be obese.

Some hormones or medications would change people's eating habits and lifestyles. Medicine may slow the burning of calories, increase appetite, or cause the body to hold extra water. People may eat more when they suffer from emotional stress. The older people grow, the more muscle people lose. Then the body burns calories more slowly and more calories store in the body.

appetite /ˈæprtaɪt/ n. 食欲

Being obese would increase the risks to many diseases as follows:

- Hypertension (high blood pressure);
- Osteoarthritis (a degeneration of cartilage and its underlying bone within a joint);
- Type 2 diabetes;
- Coronary heart disease;
- Stroke;
- Gallbladder disease;
- Sleep apnea and respiratory problems;
- Some cancers (endometrial, breast, and colon).

osteoarthritis /ˌɒstiəʊɑːˈθraitis/ n. 骨关节炎
degeneration /dɪˌdʒenəˈreɪʃ ən/ n. 恶化
cartilage /ˈkɑːtilidʒ/ n. 软骨
gallbladder /ɡɔːlˌblædə/ n. 胆囊
apnea /ˈæpniə/ n. 无呼吸，呼吸暂停
endometrial /endʌˈmetriəl/ adj. 子宫内膜的

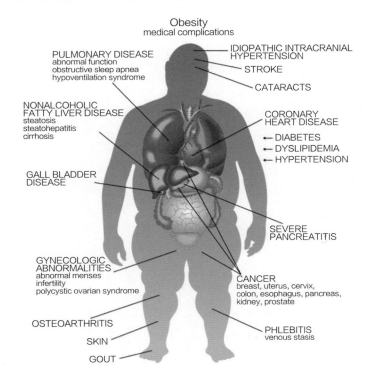

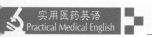

However, obese people lose 5 to 10 percent weight can prevent the risk of suffering from those diseases.

(517 words)

Text C

Stress

A decent coated white-collar may tell her friends gracefully: "Those days I feel depressed," which shocks her friends, "because the job imposes me great stress."

Lots of studies have been carried out on stress. What is stress? Stress is a word coined by Hans Selye in 1936, who defined it as "the non-specific response of the body to any demand for change". Others defined it as a feeling that occurred when the body reacted to changes. Dictionaries defined it as "physical, mental, or emotional strain or tension" or "a condition or feeling experienced when a person perceives that demands exceed the personal and social resources the individual is able to mobilize". In medical science, stress is a disruption of homeostasis through physical and psychological ways.

perceive /pə'si:v/ *vt.* 察觉
mobilize /'məubɪlaɪz/ *vt.* 调动

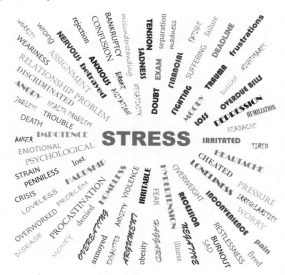

Accordingly, when a person responses to stress, there are changes in emotion, mental and physical status. Medical science could give the primary causes of stressful events by stimulating the nervous system and some hormones. And some physical alterations would handle the pressure effectively. The hypothalamus sends off signs to the adrenal glands to produce more adrenaline and cortisol, subsequently entering into the bloodstream. These hormones would speed up heart rate, breathing rate, blood pressure, and metabolism. Blood vessels open larger. Pupils dilate. Livers release more stored glucose into the bloodstream. Sweat produces. If short time stress is not great, it can help the individual cope with some emergency events, enhancing the individual's ability to perform well. While excessive stress response can cause some problems when it overreacts and fails to reset properly.

hypothalamus /ˌhaɪpəˈθæləməs/ n. 下丘脑
adrenal /əˈdriːnl/ adj. 肾上腺的
cortisol /ˈkɔːtisɒl/ n. 皮质醇

overreact /ˌəʊvərɪˈækt/ vi. 反应过度

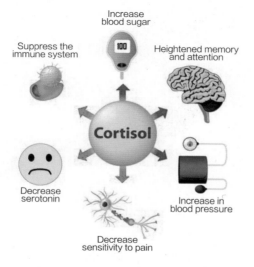

Living in a rapid working-space society, individuals should not contradict stress but can learn to adapt to and live with it. There are some ways can help people deal with stress.

contradict /ˌkɒntrəˈdɪkt/ vt. 否认⋯⋯的真实性

First of all, keep an eye on the symptoms of stress. Stress firstly has an impact on the inner emotions, causing the individual to feel anxious, panic, oppressed, or excessively worried. Then the individual may be irritable to everything and distracted from their work or become self-absorbed. If stress has not been taken under control, and the level increases over a long time, the individual would feel fatigued, upset in the stomach, headache, pain in the chest, hard sleeping, even nausea and vomiting.

distract /dɪˈstrækt/ vt. 使分心

Secondly, know how to control it. Stress is coming with new

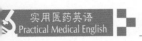

changes or challenges. Take a review at the schedule. It's wise to omit those least important matters and make the best option. Set up a realistic expectation for professional achievements. Get enough and good night sleep.

Finally, try to learn more about the causes. Both negative and positive events can lead to stress. When a sign of stress represents, try to detect the leading problems: work, study, family, society, lifestyle, and environment. If you cannot give up the matter totally, you'd better make sure that you must slow down your space while handling the event.

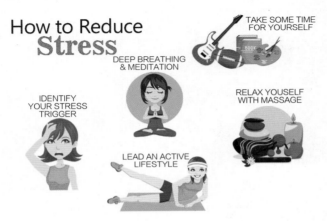

It is known that people with great stress have a tendency to take up unhealthy behaviors or habits. Therefore, stress can put health on risk. Stress comes in various forms, and it affects people of all ages. Time and space are the best recipes for stress.

(525 words)

Exercises

Task 1   Oral Practice

Direction: One student interprets the meaning of one word, and another student or other students try to guess the exact word. The game can be played in groups or pairs.

hospital	medical record	pregnancy	health	fat	body fluid
water	gene	medicine	heart rate	blood vessel	habit

Task 2   Vocabulary Exercise

Direction: Match the words or phrases with similar meaning in the two columns.

A	B
1. fatigue	a. too heavy and fat
2. hormone	b. having a baby growing inside her body
3. overweight	c. a part of a cell in a living thing that controls what it looks like, how it grows, and how it develops
4. pregnancy	d. very great tiredness
5. obesity	e. having insufficient air
6. apnea	f. a chemical substance produced by your body that influences its growth, development, and condition
7. gene	g. the general condition of body and how healthy you are
8. appetite	h. a natural form of sugar that exists in fruit
9. health	i. a desire for food
10. glucose	j. very fat in a way that is unhealthy

Task 3   Reading Comprehension

Direction: Answer the following questions according to Text A and Text B.

1. Do overweight and obesity have the same meaning? If not, what is the difference between them?
2. How does a person control living and working habits to avoid obesity?
3. Can rich living materials offer necessary happiness to people?
4. How and when does stress present?
5. Does stress always a bad thing?

Task 4   Translation

Direction: Put the passage into Chinese with the help of your dictionary.

When a client is admitted into hospital for treatment, his/her discharge plan begins. The client's requirements and wishes, family wishes, career and family circumstances will be taken into consideration. And the client can get the best support from his/her family and working unit. Normally, the client will be informed the date

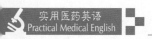

one or two days in advance when he/she is well enough to go back home. Of course, the date mainly depends on how quick the client's health improves and how much support he/she can get at home. So it's important for the client to take time to estimate the needs met at home before being discharged from the hospital.

Task 5　Prefixes, Suffixes and Roots

Direction: Learn the prefixes, suffixes or roots in the table and then choose the best answers.

Diseases（疾病）（一）

汉语 / 英语	常用词根	例　词
异常 abnormal	dys-	dysplasia 发育异常；dyspepsia 消化不良；dyspnea 呼吸困难；dysuria 排尿困难；dysfunction 机能失调
不良 bad	mal-	maladaptive 不适应的；malformation 畸形；malfunction 功能障碍；malnutrition 营养不良
慢 slow	brady-	bradypnea 呼吸过慢；bradycardia 心动过缓
快 rapid	tachy-	tachycardia 心动过速；tachypnea 呼吸急促；tachymeter 速度计；tachyuria 排尿急促
扩张 dilation	-cele	omphalocele 脐突出；hydrocele 积水；bronchocele 支气管囊肿；hematocele 血肿
发炎 inflammation	-itis	cholecystitis 胆囊炎；nephritis 肾炎；neuritis 神经炎；myocarditis 心肌炎；phlebitis 静脉炎
出血 bleeding	-rrhagia -staxis	colonorrhagia 结肠出血；cystorrhagia 膀胱出血 enterostaxis 肠渗血；bronchostaxis 支气管出血
溢出 discharge	-rrhea	diarrhea 腹泻；glycorrhea 糖溢；gastrorrhea 胃液溢出；hemorrhea 大出血
溶解 dissolving	-lysis	hydrolysis 水解；hemolysis 溶血；proteolytic 蛋白水解的；bacteriolysis 溶菌作用
嗜好 like	-philia	hydrophilia 亲水性；pharmacophilia 嗜药性
恐惧 fear	-phobia	hydrophobia 恐水病；aerophobia 高空恐惧症；carcinomatophobia 癌病恐怖
下垂 dropping	-ptosis	gastroptosis 胃下垂；nephroptosis 肾下垂；gastroenteroptosis 胃肠下垂；cardioptosis 心下垂
病毒 virus	viro-	virocytology 病毒细胞学；virogene 病毒基因；viromembrane 病毒膜；virostatic 病毒抑制药

1. The Chinese meaning for "dysuria" is _____.

    A. 排尿困难   B. 发育异常   C. 消化不良   D. 呼吸困难

2. Fill in the blank with the combining part for the medical term " 心动过缓 ": _____ cardia.

    A.tachy-   B. brady-   C. dys-   D. mal-

3. The Chinese meaning for "tachypnea" is_____.

    A. 心动过速   B. 心动过缓   C. 呼吸急促   D. 呼吸过慢

4. The English term for " 结肠出血 " is _____.

    A. bronchostaxis   B. enterostaxis

    C. cystorrhagia   D. colonorrhagia

5. The English term for " 支气管囊肿 " is _____.

    A. omphalocele   B. hydrocele

    C. hematocele   D. bronchocele

6. The word which has nothing to do with "inflammation" is _____.

    A. hepatitis   B. gastritis   C. gastroptosis   D. nephritis

7. The correct spelling for the word " 心肌炎 " is _____.

    A. bronchitis   B. myocarditis   C. phlebitis   D. cholecystitis

8. The following words have the meaning of virus except_____.

    A. bacteriolysis   B. virocytology   C. viromembrane   D. virogene

9. Which word has the meaning of " 胃肠下垂 "?

    A. Gastroenteroptosis.   B. Gastroptosis.

    C. Nephroptosis.   D. Cardioptosis.

10. The following words have the meaning of speeding except_____.

    A. tachycardia   B. bradypnea

    C. tachypnea   D. tachyuria

Task 6   Practical Writing

Direction: Read the following practical writing samples carefully and then design a similar nursing record and a medical face sheet by yourself.

Sample 1

A Nursing Record

A nursing record involves five parts: the cover, the planning sheets, the recording

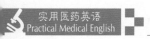

sheets, the summary sheets, and the discharge planning sheets.

- **The cover**

General illness history and treatment planning are put on the cover.

General illness history: the time of illness onset, primary symptoms, acute or chronic, examination and treatment, causes to be hospitalized

Treatment planning: treatment principles

- **The planning sheets**

This part includes date, problems, implementations and evaluation.

Problems Symptoms or discomforts resulted from physical, psychological or social factors can be solved or partly solved through nursing measurements. Causes that are definite and can affect nursing should be written down. For instance, edema in legs is caused by dysfunction of the heart.

Implementations Measurements used to improve health and relief pain

Evaluation To record generally and actually the patient's experience and examination results.

- **The recording sheets**

It is the first-hand information to reflect nursing work and disease alterations, and is not a copy of a doctor's medical record. Details are: 1) signals of illness change, vital signs, expression on the face, complaints, special treatment and positive out-comings of special examination; 2) improvements of disease; 3) reactions to treatment and nursing practices; 4) quantity and quality of sleep, diet, ventilation; 5) psychological condition and emotions; 6) major idea and analyzing content of the head nurse or chief nurse on morning visiting; 7) shifting records; 8) nursing summing-up of phases for the long-term hospitalized patient.

- **The summary sheets**

To record the major nursing problems, measurements of nursing and therapy and their effects in general terms, and to induce experiences and lessons.

- **The discharge planning sheets**

According to the mental health and illness improvements, direct the patient to estimate the needs after leaving the hospital and adapt to the life away from health care professionals. Those points should be included: diet and nutrition, activity and rest, medication, exercise, mental health, and follow up visiting.

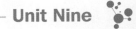

Sample 2

Medical Face Sheet

ACTIVE MEDICAL PROBLEMS

1. _____
2. _____
3. _____
4. _____
5. _____
6. _____
7. _____
8. _____

PAST HISTORY
A. Acute hospitalizations since admission to JHA

	Diagnoses	Month/Year
1.	_____	___ / ___
2.	_____	___ / ___
3.	_____	___ / ___
4.	_____	___ / ___

B. Major surgical procedures before admission to JHA

	Procedure	Year
1.	_____	_____
2.	_____	_____
3.	_____	_____
4.	_____	_____

C. Allergies

1. _____
2. _____

NEUROPSYCHIATRIC STATUS

A. Dementia
   If present: ___Absent ___Present

   ___Alzheimer's ___Mixed
   ___Multi–infarct ___Uncertain/Other

B. Psychiatric/behavioral disorders
   1. _____
   2. _____

C. Usual mental status
   ___Alert, oriented, follows simple instructions
   ___Alert, disoriented, but can follow simple directions
   ___Alert, disoriented, cannot follow simple directions
   ___Not alert (lethargic, comatose)

D. Most recent Mini Mental State Score
   ___/30 (Date____/____/____)

FUNCTIONAL STATUS

A. Ambulation
   ___Unassisted
   ___With cane
   ___With walker
   ___Unable
   Transfer ___Ind ___Dep

B. Continence

	Cont	Inc
Urine	___	___
Stool	___	___

C. Basic ADL

	Ind	Dep
Bathing	___	___
Dressing	___	___
Grooming	___	___
Feeding	___	___

D. Vision
   ___Adequate for regular print
   ___Impaired–can see large print
   ___Highly impaired–but can get around
   ___Severely impaired–has difficulty getting around

E. Hearing
   ___Adequate
   ___Minimal difficulty
   ___Hears only w/amplifier
   ___Highly impaired–no useful hearing

TREATMENT STATUS (See treatment Status Sheet Note Date___/___/___)

___Full code   ___DNR   ___DNR, do no hospitalize   ___No tube feeding

This form completed by_____ Date___/___/___

UNIT TEN

Learning Objectives

After studying this unit, you will be able to:

- ❑ Know some common expressions about the first aid kit;
- ❑ Enlarge your vocabulary related to a vaccination list and drug facts;
- ❑ Know how to administer medication;
- ❑ Talk about intravenous therapy;
- ❑ Know something about mental health, coronary heart disease and hypertension;
- ❑ Know some prefixes, suffixes or roots of medical terms about common diseases;
- ❑ Write a medical paper abstract and a medical history.

Part 1   Pictures and Charts

Warming-up: Look at the following pictures, talk about them and then finish the task.

Picture 1

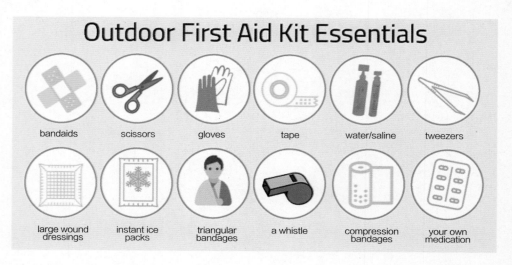

Picture 2

Vaccination List			
Age of the Vaccine Accepter	Name of the Vaccine	Time	Fee
24 hours after birth	Hepatitis B vaccine	1st	free
0 month old	Bacillus Calmette-guerin		free
1 month old	Hepatitis B vaccine	2nd	free
2 months old	Oral Polio Vaccine	1st	free
3 months old	Oral Polio Vaccine	2nd	free
	DPT	1st	free
4 months old	Oral Polio Vaccine	3rd	free
	DPT	2nd	free
5 months old	DPT	3rd	free
6 months old	Hepatitis B Vaccine	3rd	free
	Epidemic Encephalitis Vaccine	1st	free
8 months old	Measles Vaccine	1st	free
	Japanese Encephalitis	1st	free
9 months old	Epidemic Encephalitis Vaccine	2nd	free
18 months old	DPT	4th	free
	Measles Vaccine	2nd	free
2 years old	Japanese Encephalitis	2nd	free
3 years old	Epidemic Encephalitis Vaccine	3nd	free
4 years old	Oral Polio Vaccine	4th	free
6 years old	Epidemic Encephalitis Vaccine	4th	free
	Japanese Encephalitis	3rd	free
	Tetanus and Pertussis Vaccine	1st	free
16 year old	Tetanus and Pertussis Vaccine	2nd	free
	Recommended Vaccine		
after 1 year old	Hepatitis A Vaccine		
after 1 year old	Varicella Vaccine		
after 2 years old and adult	Pneumonia Vaccine		

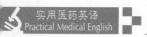
Picture 3

Drug Facts

Active ingredient (in each tablet)   Purpose
Chlorpheniramine maleate 2 mg .... Antihistamine

Uses temporarity retieves these symptoms due to hay fever or other upper respiratory allergies:
■ sneezing   ■ runny nose   ■itchy, watery eyes   ■itchy throat

Warnings
Ask a doctor betore use if you have
■ glaucorna   ■ a breathing problem such as emphysema or chronic bronchitis
■ trouble urinating due to an entarged prostate gtand

Ask a doctor or pharmacist before use if you are taiding tranquilizers or sedatives

When using this product
■ You may get drowsy   ■ avoid aicoholic drinks
■ alcohol, sedatives, and tranquilizers may increase drowsiness
■ be careful when driving a motor vehicle or operating machinery
■ excitability may occur. especially in children

If pregnant or breast-feeding, ask a health prolessional before use.
Keep out of reach of children. In case of overdose, get medical help or contact a Poison Control Center right away.

Directions

aduits and children 12 years and over	take 2 tablets every 4 to 6 hours; not more than 12 tablets in 24 hours
children 6 years to under 12 years	take 1 tablet every 4 to 6 hours; not more than 6 tablets in 24 hours
children under 6 years	ask a doctor

Other information store at 20~25℃(68~77℉)   ■ protect from excessive moisture

Inactive ingredients D&C yellow no. 10. tactose, magnesium stearate. microcrystalline cellulose. pregelatinized starch

Task: Match the words in the left column with the explanations in the right column.

1. vaccine	A. an excessive and dangerous dose of a drug
2. epidemic	B. a widespread occurrence of an infectious disease in a community at a particular time
3. drowsy	C. a substance injected into the body to cause it to produce antibodies and so provide immunity against a disease
4. overdose	D. sleepy
5. first-aid kit	E. kit consisting of a set of bandages and medicines for giving first aid

Part 2 Listening and Speaking

Conversation A

Administration of Medication

(The nurse is telling her patient how to take the medicine.)

Nurse: Good morning, Mr. Bill! Are you feeling better today?

Patient: No. I have pain in my wound and I can't sleep well.

Nurse: The doctor has prescribed something to ease your pain and improve your sleep.

Patient: Thanks!

Nurse: Are you allergic to any type of medication?

DR. OZ'S PRESCRIPTION FOR OVER-THE-COUNTER DRUGS
OBEY DIRECTIONS
TALK TO YOUR PHARMACIST
CHOOSE LOWEST DOSE FIRST

Patient: I don't know exactly. I have never been allergic to any medicine before.

Nurse: The medicine in the box is for oral use. In case of any complications, just tell us.

oral /ˈɔːrəl/
adj. 口的，口腔的

Patient: I will. Could you tell me how to take this medicine?

Nurse: You should take it with boiled water before meals, three times a day, two tablets each time.

tablet /ˈtæblɪt/ *n.* 药片

Patient: Is the medicine in the bottle also for internal use?

Nurse: No, it is only for external use. Apply the ointment in the bottle to your wound whenever you have pain.

external /ɪkˈstɜːnl/
adj. 外用的
ointment /ˈɔɪntmənt/
n. 药膏

Patient: How much should I use each time?

Nurse: You can follow the directions on the label.

Patient: Ok. I remember I took some red pills yesterday. Should I stop using them now?

Nurse: Yes. The function of those pills is to treat inflammation. According to Doctor Li, you needn't take them anymore.

Patient: Why not?

Nurse: Because your infection has already improved a lot. What's more, drugs have some adverse side-effects to a greater or lesser degree. Long-term and constant use of them will affect your stomach.

adverse /ˈædvɜːs/
adj. 不利的

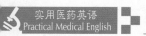

Patient: I see.

Nurse: By the way, make sure that you eat plenty of fruits and vegetables every day. That will help your bowel movements. Furthermore, sufficient intake of vitamins will speed the healing process.

Patient: I will try. Thank you for telling me so many useful things.

Nurse: You are welcome! I hope you'll recover soon!

(301 words)

Conversation B

Intravenous Therapy

Task 1: Watch episode one and fill in the missing words referring to the original text. Then check your writing against the original.

Nurse: Morning, Miss Susan. I am Mary. I will be looking after you today.

Patient: Morning, Mary. Pleased to meet you. How does my _____ culture look? I can't handle the pain anymore. Today I have to go to the _____ more often.

Nurse: Your urine culture indicated you have a urinary tract _____. And Doctor Wilson prescribed intravenous _____ according to your sensitivity test.

Patient: You mean you will give me an IV right now?

Nurse: Yes, if you are ready.

Patient: Ok. Do I need to take the _____ _____ first?

Nurse: No need. But you can go to the bathroom first and I will come back later.

Patient: Sure. See you later.

Task 2: Watch episode two and complete the answers according to the questions.

1. What did the nurse do before giving the patient an IV?

The nurse checked _____ _____ first.

2. What are the steps to have an IV?

Lie down and make yourself comfortable. Hold your hand for a minute. Then _____ your hand.

3. If the patient needs help, what can he do?

Please ring this _____ _____if the patient need help.

Part 3 Reading Comprehension

Text A

Attention to Mental Health

October tenth is World Mental Health Day. This year's observance centers on the relationship between mental health and chronic physical conditions like diabetes and cancer.

observance /əb'zɜːvəns/ n.(对风俗或仪式的) 遵守

The World Health Organization says more than four hundred fifty million people suffer from poor mental health. The most common disorders are depression and schizophrenia. Mental health experts also include other disorders like drug and alcohol abuse that affect millions of people.

schizophrenia /ˌskɪtsəu'friːnɪə/ n. 精神分裂症

alcohol /'ælkəhɒl/ n. 酒精

abuse /ə'bjuːs/ n. 滥用

affect /ə'fekt/ vt. 影响

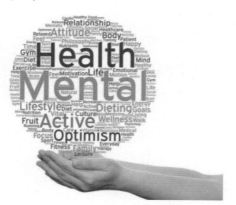

Elena Berger is with the World Federation for Mental Health. That organization, based in the United States, held the first World Mental Health Day in 1992.

Mrs. Berger says mental health problems are most severe in poor countries that lack the resources to deal with them.

She says,"It's an enormous issue. The World Health Organization is highlighting mental health as a neglected issue. In developing countries, a huge number of people, up to eighty-five percent, don't have access to any form of mental health treatment. There are huge staffing needs. There are no services. And there's a lot of stigma in a lot of societies about being mentally ill."

enormous /ɪ'nɔːməs/ adj. 巨大的

access /'ækses/ n. 通道

stigma /'stɪgmə/ n. 耻辱

Experts say about half of all mental health problems first appear

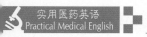
before the age of fifteen. The countries with the highest percentages of young people are in the developing world. That means they are also the countries with the poorest levels of mental health resources.

The World Health Organization says many low- and middle-income countries have only one child psychiatrist for every one to four million people.

Worldwide, depression is the leading mental health problem and a leading cause of disability. In two thousand two, the World Health Organization estimated that more than one hundred fifty-four million people suffered from depression.

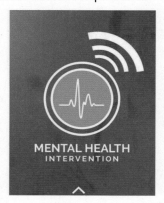

But Mrs. Berger says other kinds of diseases often get more attention.

She says,"People are more focused on communicable diseases and not paying enough attention to the amount of disability from mental health conditions. And these are real disabilities where people are not able to work to their full capacity, can't earn an income. And there's a big impact on families as well."

Mrs. Berger says her organization and the World Health Organization are pushing to have governments include mental health care in their development goals. She says this could greatly improve the availability of treatment and services worldwide.

She says,"People with mental and psychosocial disabilities would be recognized as vulnerable groups that need special support, and who need to be included in society, and not excluded and ignored as is often the case at the present time."

(422 words)

percentage /pəˈsentɪdʒ/ n. 百分比

communicable /kəˈmjuːnɪkəbl/ adj. 可传染的

capacity /kəˈpæsɪtɪ/ n. 能力
availability /əˌveɪləˈbɪlɪtɪ/ n. 有效性
psychosocial /ˌsaɪkəʊˈsəʊʃəl/ adj. 社会心理的
vulnerable /ˈvʌlnərəbəl/ adj. 易受伤害的

exclude /ɪksˈkluːd/ vt. 排斥

Text B

Coronary Heart Disease

The heart pumps blood around your body and beats approximately 70 times a minute. After the blood leaves the heart, it goes to your lungs where it picks up oxygen. The oxygen-rich blood returns to your heart and is then pumped to the organs of your body through a network of arteries. The blood returns to your heart through veins before being pumped back to your lungs again. This process is called blood circulation.

The heart gets its own supply of blood from a network of blood vessels on the surface of your heart, called coronary arteries. Coronary heart disease is the term that describes what happens when your heart's blood supply is blocked, or interrupted, by a build-up of fatty substances in the coronary arteries.

approximately
/əprɒksɪ'mətlɪ/
adv. 大约

vein /veɪn/ *n.* 静脉
circulation /ˌsɜːkjʊ'leɪʃən/
n. 循环
vessel /'vesl/ *n.* 脉管
artery /'ɑːtərɪ/ *n.* 动脉

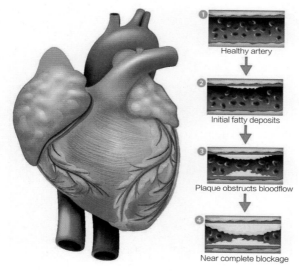

① Healthy artery

② Initial fatty deposits

③ Plaque obstructs bloodflow

④ Near complete blockage

If your coronary arteries become partially blocked, it can cause chest pain (angina). If they become completely blocked, it can cause a heart attack (myocardial infarction). Heart attacks can cause permanent damage to the heart muscle and, if not treated straight away, can be fatal. If you think that you have a heart attack, you should dial 120 for immediate medical assistance.

If you have coronary heart disease, you may experience heart palpitations. Heart palpitations occur when your heart beats

partially /'pɑːʃəlɪ/
adv. 部分地
angina /æn'dʒaɪnə/
n. 心绞痛
myocardial
/ˌmaɪəʊ'kɑːdɪəl/
adj. 心肌的
infarction /ɪn'fɑːkʃən/
n. 梗塞（梗死）形成
palpitation /ˌpælpɪ'teɪʃən/
n. 心悸

irregularly, or harder than normal. It is important to realize that heart palpitations are not necessarily linked to coronary heart disease and, if you experience them, you should not worry unduly. However, it is always best to have it checked out by your physician.

unduly /ʌnˈdjuːlɪ/
adv. 过度地

Heart failure can occur in people with coronary heart disease. The heart becomes too weak to pump blood around the body which can cause fluid to build up in the lungs, making it increasingly difficult to breathe. Heart failure can happen suddenly (acute heart failure), or gradually, over a period of time (chronic heart failure).

Your risk of developing coronary heart disease is significantly increased if you:

- Smoke;
- Have high blood pressure;
- Have a high blood cholesterol level;
- Do not take regular exercise;
- Have a thrombosis;
- Have diabetes.

cholesterol /kəˈlestərəul/
n. 胆固醇
thrombosis /θrɒmˈbəusɪs/
n. 血栓症

Coronary heart disease cannot be cured, but recent progress in the research and development of new medicines and significant improvements in surgical procedures have meant that the condition can now be managed more effectively. With the right treatment, the symptoms of coronary heart disease can be reduced, and the functioning of the heart improved.

If your blood vessels are very narrow due to a build-up of atheroma (fatty deposits), or if your symptoms cannot be controlled using medication, surgery may be needed to open up, or replace,

atheroma /ˌæθəˈrəumə/
n. 动脉粥样化

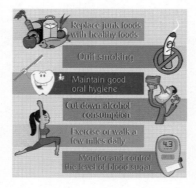

the blocked arteries. Some surgical procedures, for example, coronary artery bypass, heart transplant and laser surgery can be used to treat blocked arteries.

bypass /'baɪpɑːs/
n. 旁通管
transplant /træns'plɑːnt/
n. 移植

The best way to prevent coronary heart disease is to make sure that your low-density lipoprotein (LDL) level is low and that your high-density lipoprotein (HDL) is high. There are a number of ways you can do this including:

- Eat a healthy, balanced diet;
- Be more physically active;
- Give up smoking;
- Reduce your alcohol consumption;

consumption
/kən'sʌmpʃən/ n. 消费

- Keep your blood pressure under control;
- Keep your diabetes under control;
- Take any medication that is prescribed for you.

(539 words)

Text C

Hypertension

High blood pressure, termed "hypertension", is a condition that afflicts almost 1 billion people worldwide and is a leading cause of morbidity and mortality. Many people are not even aware they are hypertensive. Therefore, this disease is sometimes called the "silent killer". This disease is usually asymptomatic until the damaging effects of hypertension (such as stroke, myocardial infarction, renal dysfunction, visual problems, etc.) are observed.

hypertension
/ˌhaɪpə'tenʃən/
n. 高血压
afflict /ə'flɪkt/ vt. 折磨

asymptomatic
/ˌeɪsɪmptə'mætɪk/
adj. 无症状的
stroke /strəuk / n. 中风
dysfunction /dɪs'fʌŋkʃən/
n. 功能紊乱

Hypertensive is defined as an abnormal elevation of blood pressure. Both systolic and diastolic pressure values are important to note. According to the latest U.S. national diagnosis guidelines, the following values represent different stages of hypertension.

systolic /ˌsɪs'tɒlɪk/
adj. 心脏收缩的
diastolic /ˌdaɪə'stɒlɪk/
adj. 心脏舒张的
value /'væljuː/ n. (数) 值

For 90% to 95% of patients presenting with hypertension, the cause is unknown. This condition is called primary (or essential) hypertension. The remaining 5% to 10% of hypertensive patients have hypertension that results secondarily from renal disease,

primary /'praɪmərɪ/
adj. 原发性的

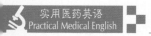
KNOW YOUR BLOOD PRESSURE
—AND WHAT TO DO ABOUT IT

— By AMERICAN HEART ASSOCIATION NEWS —

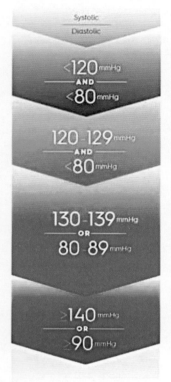

The newest guidelines for hypertension:

NORMAL BLOOD PRESSURE
*Recommendations: Healthy lifestyle choices and yearly checks.

ELEVATED BLOOD PRESSURE
*Recommendations: Healthy lifestyle changes, reassessed in 3–6 months.

HIGH BLOOD PRESSURE / STAGE 1
*Recommendations: 10–year heart disease and stroke risk assessment. If less than 10% risk, lifestyle changes, reassessed in 3–6 months. If higher, lifestyle changes and medication with monthly follow–ups until BP controlled.

HIGH BLOOD PRESSURE / STAGE 2
*Recommendations: Lifestyle changes and 2 different classes of medicine, with monthly follow–ups until BP is controlled.

endocrine disorders, or other identifiable causes. This form of hypertension is called secondary hypertension.

A hypertensive crisis is a severe increase in blood pressure that can lead to a stroke. Extremely high blood pressure damages blood vessels. The heart may not be able to maintain adequate circulation of blood. A hypertensive crisis is divided into two categories: urgent and emergency. Signs and symptoms of an urgent hypertensive crisis may include elevated blood pressure, severe headache, severe anxiety, and shortness of breath. During a hypertensive emergency, you may experience life-threatening signs and symptoms, such as pulmonary edema, brain swelling or bleeding, heart attack stroke.

In most cases of hypertension, doctors can't point to the exact cause. But several things are known to raise blood pressure, including being very overweight, drinking too much alcohol, having

identifiable /aɪˈdentɪfaɪəbl/
adj. 可以确认的
secondary /ˈsekəndərɪ/
adj. 继发性的

category /ˈkætɪgərɪ/
n. 种类

a family history of high blood pressure, eating too much salt, and getting older. Your blood pressure may also rise if you are not very active, you don't eat enough potassium and calcium.

potassium /pə'tæsjəm/ *n.* 钾

High blood pressure doesn't usually cause symptoms. Most people don't know they have it until they go to the doctor for some other reason. Without treatment, high blood pressure can damage the heart, brain, kidneys, or eyes. This damage causes problems like coronary artery disease, stroke, and kidney failure. Very high blood pressure can cause headaches, vision problems, nausea, and vomiting.

Treatment depends on how high your blood pressure is, whether you have other health problems such as diabetes, and whether any organs have already been damaged. Your doctor will also consider how likely you are to develop other diseases, especially heart disease. Most people with hypertension are treated with antihypertensive medications. Hypertension is also commonly treated with drugs that decrease cardiac output. Vasodilator drugs, which decrease systemic vascular resistance, are also used to treat hypertension.

antihypertensive /'ænti,haipə'tensiv/ *adj.* 抗高血压的
cardiac /'kɑːdiæk/ *adj.* 心脏的
vasodilator /,væsəudai'leitə/ *adj.* 血管扩张的
systemic /sis'temik/ *adj.* 全身的
vascular /'væskjulə/ *adj.* 血管的

You can help lower your blood pressure by making healthy changes in your lifestyle. If those lifestyle changes don't work, you may also need to take pills. Lifestyle changes you can make to help prevent high blood pressure include:

- Lose extra weight;
- Eat less salt;
- Exercise;
- Limit alcohol;
- Get 3,500 mg of potassium in your diet every day. Fresh, unprocessed whole foods have the most potassium. These foods include meat, fish, nonfat and low-fat dairy products, and many fruits and vegetables.

unprocessed /,ʌn'prəusest/ *adj.* 未被加工的

(546 words)

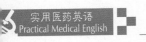

Exercises

Task 1　Oral Practice

Direction: Read aloud the following words or phrases and try to learn them by heart. Then one student will ask "where is your…?" or "please show me your…!" The other students should act with proper body movements or gestures. The student who acts most correctly or promptly will be the winner. The game can be played in groups or pairs.

shoulder	elbow	armpit	joint	knee	lower limb
neck	forehead	wrist	nail	palm	stomach
throat	upper arm	chin	forefinger	back	rib
lung	liver	chest	heart	belly	cheek

Task 2　Vocabulary Exercise

Direction: Match the words or phrases with similar meaning in the two columns.

<table>
<tr><td align="center">A</td><td align="center">B</td></tr>
<tr><td>1. hypertension</td><td>a. additional</td></tr>
<tr><td>2. approximately</td><td>b. to obstruct</td></tr>
<tr><td>3. vision</td><td>c. to raise</td></tr>
<tr><td>4. systemic</td><td>d. to trouble</td></tr>
<tr><td>5. elevate</td><td>e. fatty deposits</td></tr>
<tr><td>6. category</td><td>f. about</td></tr>
<tr><td>7. afflict</td><td>g. high blood pressure</td></tr>
<tr><td>8. block</td><td>h. sight</td></tr>
<tr><td>9. atheroma</td><td>i. all over the body</td></tr>
<tr><td>10. extra</td><td>j. kind</td></tr>
</table>

Task 3　Reading Comprehension

Direction: Decide whether the following statements are true or false according to Text A and Text B.

1. If your coronary arteries become only partially blocked, it can cause myocardial infarction.

2. Heart palpitations occur when your heart beats irregularly, or harder than normal.

3. Some surgical procedures, for example, coronary artery bypass, heart transplant and laser surgery can be used to treat blocked arteries.

4. An urgent hypertensive crisis may include life-threatening signs and symptoms, such as pulmonary edema, brain swelling or bleeding, heart attack, stroke.

5. Obtaining enough potassium in your daily diet can help prevent high blood pressure.

Task 4　Translation

Direction: Put the passage into Chinese with the help of your dictionary.

A number of different tests are used to diagnose heart-related problems including:

1) Coronary angiogram: It provides information about the blood pressure inside your heart, and how well the chambers and valves are working.

2) Electrocardiogram (ECG): It records the rhythm and electrical activity of your heart and can sometimes show if a person has had a heart attack.

3) Magnetic Resonance Imaging (MRI): It can be used to produce detailed pictures of your heart, and blood vessels, and can measure the flow of blood through your heart and major arteries.

4) Electrophysiological testing: It can help diagnose abnormal heart rhythms, and can show whether they are being effectively controlled with certain medicines. It can also identify whether the abnormal heart rhythm is causing palpitations.

Task 5　Prefixes, Suffixes and Roots

Direction: Learn the prefixes, suffixes or roots in the table and then choose the best answers.

Diseases（疾病）（二）

汉语 / 英语	常用词根	例　词
肿瘤 tumour	onc(h)/o-	oncogene 致癌或瘤基因；oncology 肿瘤学；oncocyte 肿瘤细胞；oncogen 致肿瘤物
	-oma	myofibroma 肌纤维瘤；melanoma 黑色素瘤
疾病 disease	path/o-	pathogen 病原体；histopathology 组织病理学；pathoanatomy 病理解剖学
	-pathy	gastropathy 胃病；neuropathy 神经病；nephropathy 肾病

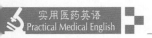

(Continued)

汉语 / 英语	常用词根	例　词
脓 pus	py/o-	pyocyst 脓囊肿；pyorrhea 脓漏；pyogenesis 化脓；pyuria 脓尿
发烧 fever	pyr/o- pyret/o-	pyrogenous 高热所产生的；pyrexia 发烧；hyperpyrecia 高烧 pyretology 热病学；pyretic 发热的；pyretolysis 退烧
硬化 hardening	scler/o-	sclerosis 硬化症；arteriosclerosis 动脉硬化症；sclerometer 硬度计；scleroderma 硬皮病
软化 softening	malac(i)/o-	malacic 软化的；splenomalacia 脾软化；aortomalacia 主动脉软化；cardiomalacia 心肌软化
狭窄 narrowing	steno/o-	esophagostenosis 食管狭窄；angiostenosis 血管狭窄；enterostenosis 肠道狭窄；cardiostenosis 心腔狭窄
肿大 dilation	-ectasis megalo- -megaly	bronchiectasis 支气管扩张；lymphadenectasis 淋巴结肿大 megalocardia 心肥大； hepatomegaly 肝肿大；splenomegaly 脾脏肿大； hepatolienomegaly 肝脾肿大

1. The Chinese meaning for "melanoma" is _____.

    A. 黑色素瘤　　　　B. 肌纤维瘤　　　　C. 肿瘤细胞　　　　D. 致癌基因

2. Fill in the blank with the combining part for the medical term " 神经病 ": neuro-_____.

    A.oma　　　　　　B. pathy　　　　　C. ectasis　　　　　D. itis

3. The Chinese meaning for "arteriosclerosis" is_____.

    A. 硬皮病　　　　　B. 硬化症　　　　　C. 主动脉硬化　　　D. 主动脉软化

4. The English term for " 脾软化 " is _____.

    A. arteriosclerosis　　　　　　　　B. cardiomalacia

    C. aortomalacia　　　　　　　　　D. splenomalacia

5. The English term for " 肠道狭窄 " is _____.

    A. angiostenosis　　　　　　　　　B. cardiostenosis

    C. esophagostenosis　　　　　　　D. enterostenosis

6. The word which has nothing to do with "enlargement" is _____.

    A. angiostenosis　　　　　　　　　B. cardiostenosis

    C. hepatomegaly　　　　　　　　　D. enterostenosis

7. The correct spelling for the word " 支气管扩张 " is _____.

    A. bronchitis　　　　　　　　　　B. bronchiectasis

    C. bronchoscope　　　　　　　　　D. bronchopneumonia

8. The following words have the meaning of fever except_____.

    A. pathogen   B. pyrexia   C. hyperpyrexia   D. pyretolysis

9. Which word has the meaning of "脓囊肿"?

    A. Pyuria.   B. Pyogenesis.

    C. Pyocyst.   D. Pyorrhea.

10. The following words have the meaning of disease except_____.

    A. gastropathy   B. glucometer   C. neuropathy   D. nephropathy

Task 6   Practical Writing

Direction: Read the following practical writing samples carefully and then write a similar paper abstract and a medical history by yourself.

Sample 1

Paper Abstract

An Investigation, Assessment and Analysis of the Nursing Quality Control Work

[Abstract] Purpose: To promote the quality control awareness of the nursing personnel, acquire enough information about the quality control work in the hospital, adjust the hospital's management model, activate the nursing personnel to participate in quality control work, and thus improve nursing quality constantly. Method: Questionnaires are devised, handed out, collected and analyzed to assess the quality control and management system in the hospital. Result: 82.83% personnel investigated agree that the existing quality control system in the hospital runs effectively. 92.92% have a positive attitude toward the principles of justice, fairness and publicity in quality control work. 37.37% think the punishment measures from the nursing department are rational. 42.42% agree that the quality control frequency is reasonable. Conclusion: According to the investigation statistic, the nursing department has comprehensively gathered various viewpoints and attitudes from nursing personnel in the hospital so that quality control management style can be adjusted, the quality control model can be constantly bettered and the nursing quality can be improved.

Key Words: Nursing; Quality Control; Assessment; Analysis

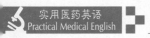

Sample 2

A Method to Take a Medical History
— "SAMPLE PQRST"

S—Symptoms

A—Allergies

M—Medicine taken

P—Past history of similar events

L—Last meal

E—Events leading up to illness or injury

P—Provocation/Position (what brought symptoms on/where is pain located)

Q—Quality (sharp, dull, crushing, etc.)

R—Radiation (does pain travel)

S—Severity/Symptoms associated with (on a scale of 1 to 10/ what other symptoms occur)

T—Timing/Triggers (occasional, constant, intermittent/only when I do this activity...)

Example:

1) 21 y/o male c/o sore throat. No known allergies. Taking no meds. Has approx.

2) Sore throats per year. Eating and drinking normally. Was fine until yesterday morning when woke up with a sore throat. Denies fevers, chills, sweats, shortness of breath,& headache.

APPENDICES

1. Commonly Used Medical Terms

1) 内科常用词

acute upper respiratory tract infection	急性上呼吸道感染
antiphospholipid	抗磷脂
behcet disease	白塞氏病
boarding hypertension	临界高血压
bronchial asthma	支气管哮喘
chronic bronchitis	慢性支气管炎
chronic pulmonary heart disease	慢性肺源性心脏病
churg-strauss syndrome	变应性肉芽肿性血管炎
cirrhosis of liver	肝硬化
discoid rash	盘状红斑
duodenal ulcers	十二指肠溃疡
essential (primary) hypertension	原发性高血压
gastric ulcer (GU)	胃溃疡
giant cell arteritis	巨细胞动脉炎
hepatic encephalopathy (HE)	肝性脑病
hypertension emergency	高血压急症
intestinal tuberculosis	肠结核
kashin-beck disease	大骨节病
legionnaires pneumonia	军团菌肺炎
lobar pneumonia	大叶肺炎
lung abscess	肺脓肿
malignant hypertension	恶性高血压
molar rash	蝶形红斑
mycoplasmal pneumonia	支原体肺炎

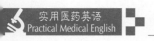
nephritic syndrome (NS)	肾病综合征
osteoarthritis	骨性关节炎
peptic ulcer	消化性溃疡
pericardial effusion	心包积液
pericarditis	心包炎
pleural effusion	胸腔积液
polyarteritis nodosa	结节性多动脉炎
primary bronchogenic carcinoma	支气管癌
primary carcinoma of the liver	肝癌
pulmonary tuberculosis	肺结核
reiter syndrome	瑞特综合征
secondary hypertension	继发性高血压
sjogren syndrome	干燥综合征
systemic sclerosis	系统性硬化病
temporal arteritis	颞动脉炎
tuberculosis peritonitis	结核性腹膜炎
ulcerative colitis (UC)	溃疡性结肠炎
vasculitis	血管炎（结节性脉管炎）
viral myocarditis	病毒性心肌炎
virus pneumonia	病毒性肺炎

2) 外科常用词

abdominal external hernia	腹外疝
acute appendicitis	急性阑尾炎
acute diffuse peritonitis	急性弥漫性腹膜炎
acute mastitis	急性乳腺炎
acute pancreatitis	急性胰腺炎
acute pyelonephritis	急性肾盂肾炎
anal fissure	肛裂
anal fistula	肛瘘
anesthesia	麻醉
angioma	血管瘤
appendicitis	阑尾炎
burn	烧伤

cancer of breast	乳腺癌
carbuncle	痈
carcinoma of colon	结肠癌
carcinoma of esophagus	食道癌
carcinoma of gallbladder	胆囊癌
carcinoma of rectum	直肠癌
carcinoma of stomach	胃癌
cerebral concussion	脑震荡
cervical spondylosis	颈椎病
cholecystitis	胆囊炎
cholecystolithiasis	胆囊结石
choledochitis	胆总管炎
choledocholithiasis	胆总管结石病
cholelithiasis	胆石症
chondroma	软骨瘤
dislocation of joint	关节脱位
intestinal fistula	肠瘘
intestinal obstruction	肠梗阻
primary lower extremity varicose veins	原发性下肢静脉曲张
pyloric obstruction	幽门梗阻

3) 妇儿科常用词

anterior fontanel	前囟
bacterial vaginosis	细菌性阴道病
bottle-feeding	人工喂养
breast cancer	乳腺癌
breast feeding	母乳喂养
breast health	乳房健康
breast self-exam	乳房自检
child care	儿童保健
defecation	排便
disease prevention	疾病预防
ectopic pregnancy	宫外孕
fallopian tube	输卵管

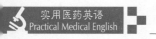

female hormones	雌激素
fetal stage	胎儿期
gynecological health	妇科健康
infant feeding	婴儿喂养
instruction of solid food	添加辅食
insufficiency of intake	摄入不足
malnutrition	缺乏营养
menopause syndrome	绝经综合征
menstrual cramps	痛经
missed or irregular periods	月经不调
mixed feeding	混合喂养
neonatal period	新生儿期
nutrition and metabolism	营养代谢
obesity in childhood	小儿肥胖
pediatrics	儿科学
pelvic examination	盆腔检查
pelvic infection	盆腔感染
planned immunity	计划免疫
posterior	后囟
pregnancy test	妊娠检查
premature labor	早产
premature	早产儿
premenstrual syndromes	月经前综合征
sexually transmitted disease	性病
summit of growth	生长高峰
term infant	足月儿
trichomoniasis	滴虫病
uterine fibroids	子宫纤维瘤
vaccination	预防接种
vaginal bleeding	阴道出血
vaginal discharge	阴道分泌物
vaginal thrush	霉菌性阴道炎
yeast infections	真菌感染

4) 五官科常用词

auricle	耳廓
choroid	脉络膜
colliery body	睫状体
conjunctiva	结膜
cornea	角膜
deciduous teeth	乳牙
epistaxis	鼻出血
eyeball	眼球
eyelid	眼睑
gum of gingival	牙龈
gustatory organ	味蕾
internal ear	内耳
iris	虹膜
lachrymal gland	泪腺
lens	晶状体
nasal bone	鼻骨
nasal bridge	鼻梁
ophthalmic	眼动脉
optic nerve	视神经
oral cavity	口腔
pulp	牙髓
retina	视网膜
sclera	巩膜
tympanic	鼓膜
visual organ	视器

5) 皮肤科常用词

acne	痤疮
atrophy	萎缩
condyloma acuminatum	尖锐湿疣
crust	痂
cyst	囊肿

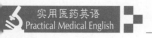

drug eruption	药疹
eczema	湿疹
erosion	糜烂
excoriation	抓痕
fissure	皲裂
gonorrhea	淋病
herpes simplex	单纯疱疹
herpes zoster	带状疱疹
impetigo	脓疱疹
macule	斑疹
neurodermatitis	神经性皮炎
papule	丘疹
pediculosis	虱病
psoriasis	银屑病
pustule	脓包
scabies	疥疮
scale	鳞屑
syphilis	梅毒
ulceration	溃疡
urethritis	尿道
urticaria	荨麻疹
wart	疣
wheal	风团炎

6) 常用护理技术用语

absolute diet (fasting)	禁食
applying cold compresses	冷敷
applying hot compresses	热敷
applying hot soaks	湿热敷
applying hot water bottles	用热水瓶
arterial transfusion	动脉输血
asepsis	无菌（法）
aspiration (suction) drainage	吸引导液（引流）
assessment	估计

assisting the patient to take a sitz bath	帮病人坐浴
balanced diet	平衡饮食
barium enema	钡灌肠
bathing	洗澡
bedmaking	整理床铺
bedsore care	褥疮护理
bladder irrigation	膀胱冲洗
bland diet	清淡饮食
blind enema	肛管排气法
blood (body fluid) precautions	血液（体液）预防措施
blood transfusion	输血
brushing the teeth	刷牙
cardiac catheterization	心导管插入术
cardiac decompression	心肺减压术
cardiopulmonary resuscitation	心肺复苏术
care of nails and feet	指甲修剪和洗脚
catheterization	导管插入术
cerebral decompression	脑减压术
changing hospital gowns	更换住院服装
chemical sterilization	化学灭菌法
cleanliness and skin care	清洁与皮肤护理
clean techniques (medical asepsis)	消毒灭菌（医学无菌）
closed drainage	关闭引流法
concomitant (concurrent) disinfection	随时（即时）消毒
contact isolation	接触隔离
continuous irrigation	连续冲洗法
contrast enema	对比灌肠
convalescent diet	恢复期饮食
counting respiration	计呼吸次数
daily care of the patient	对病人日常护理
decompression of pericardium	心包减压术
decompression of rectum	直肠减压术
decompression of spinal cord	脊髓减压术
decompression	减压（术）

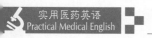

denture care	清洗假牙
diabetic diet	糖尿病饮食
dialysis	透析
diet nursing	饮食护理
direct (immediate) transfusion	直接输血
disinfection by ultraviolet light	紫外线消毒
disinfection	消毒
drainage (secretion) precautions	引流预防措施
drainage	引流（导液）
drip transfusion	滴注输血（液）
emergency care (first aid)	急救护理
emergency care for a patient during a seizure	癫痫发作急救
emergency care given to help a patient who is vomiting	呕吐患者急救
emergency care used to control hemorrhage	止血急救
endemic (intracutaneous) injection	皮内注射
endemic medication	皮内投药法
enema	灌肠
enteric precautions	肠道预防措施
epidemic medication	皮上投药法
eucaloric diet	适当热量饮食
evaluation	评价
fat-free diet	无脂饮食
feeding	喂养
fever diet	热病饮食
flossing the teeth	清牙垢
forced (forcible) feeding	强制喂养
full diet	全食或普通饮食
gastric lavage	洗胃
gastro-intestinal decompression	胃肠减压术
giving a cold (an alcohol) sponge bath	冷水（酒精）擦浴
glucose-saline infusion	葡萄糖和盐水输注
glucose infusion	葡萄糖液输注
glycerin enema	甘油灌肠
hair care	头发护理

half diet	半食
heat and cold application	冷热敷
hemodialysis	血液透析
high (low) enema	高（低）位灌肠
high-carbohydrate diet	高糖饮食
high-protein (protein-rich) diet	高蛋白饮食
high caloric diet	高热量饮食
high fat diet	高脂饮食
hospice care	临终护理
hypertonic saline injection	高渗盐水注射
hypodermatic medication	皮下投药法
hypodermic injection	皮下注射
indirect transfusion	间接输血
infusion	输液
injection	注射
integral asepsis	完全无菌
intermittent sterilization	间歇灭菌法
intervention (implementation)	措施（实施）管理
intestinal lavage	洗肠
intramuscular injection	肌肉注射
intraocular injection	眼球内注射
intrapleural injection	胸腹腔注射
intrauterine injection	子宫内注射
intubation (tube) feeding	管饲法
invalid diet	病弱者饮食
ionic medication	离子透药疗法
irrigation	冲洗
isolation	隔离
laryngeal catheterization (intubation)	喉插管术
lavage	灌洗
light diet	易消化饮食
liquid diet	流质饮食
low-protein diet	低蛋白饮食
low-residue diet	低渣饮食

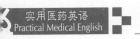

low caloric diet	低热量饮食
low fat diet	低脂饮食
magnesium sulfate enema	硫酸镁灌肠
massage	按摩
measurement of vital signs	测量生命体征
measuring (taking) blood pressure	测量血压
mediate irrigation	间接冲洗法
medication	药疗、投药、给药
morning (evening) care	晨（晚）间护理
mouth-to-mouth resuscitation	口对口复苏术
mouth-to-nose resuscitation	口对鼻复苏术
nasal feeding	鼻饲法
nasal injection	鼻内注射
nasal medication	鼻内投药法
nasogastric suctioning	鼻胃抽吸
negative pressure drainage	负压吸引法
nourishing diet	滋补饮食
nursing diagnosis	护理诊断
nursing processes	护理过程
obesity diet	肥胖饮食
open drainage	开放引流法
oral hygiene (mouth care)	口腔卫生
oral medication	口服药
orbital decompression	眼眶减压术
perineal care	会阴部护理
peritoneal dialysis	腹膜透析
peritoneal injection	腹膜腔注射
peritoneal lavage	腹膜腔灌洗
plasma transfusion	输血清
pleural lavage	胸膜腔灌洗
postmortem care	死后护理
postural drainage	体位引流法
prenatal diet	孕期饮食
protective isolation	保护性隔离

rectal feeding	直肠营养法
rectal injection	直肠注射
rectal medication	直肠投药法
regimens diet	规定食谱
respiratory isolation	呼吸道隔离
retention (non-retention) enema	保留（无保留）灌肠
retro-urethral catheterization	逆行导尿管插入术
saline infusion	盐水输注
salt-free diet	无盐饮食
shaving	刮脸
smooth (soft) diet	细（微）饮食
soapsuds enema	肥皂水灌肠
steam disinfection	蒸汽消毒
sterilization	灭菌、消毒
strict isolation	严密隔离
subconjunctival injection	结膜下注射
sublingual medication	舌下投药法
suctioning	吸气、引液
taking a radial pulse	测量桡动脉脉搏
taking axillary temperature	测量腋下温度
taking oral temperature	测量口腔温度
taking rectal temperature	测量直肠温度
terminal disinfection	终末消毒
transduodenal medication	十二指肠内投药法
turpentine enema	松节油灌肠
upper airway suctioning	上呼吸道抽吸
urethral catheterization	尿道导管插入术
urethral injection	尿道注射
vaginal drainage	阴道引流法
vaginal injection	阴道注射
vaginal irrigation	阴道冲洗
vaginal medication	阴道投药法
venous transfusion	静脉输血（液）
vesicocelomic drainage	膀胱腹腔引流

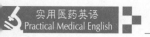

| wound suctioning | 伤口吸引 |

7) 常用护理器械

absorbent cotton	脱脂棉
adhesive plaster	胶布
alcohol burner	酒精灯
ampoule (ampule)	安瓿
anal speculum	肛门扩张器（扩肛器）
aural speculum	耳廓器（耳镜）
autoclave sterilizer (disinfector)	高压蒸汽灭菌器
automatic ventilator	自动呼吸机
bandage	绷带
bath towel	浴巾
bedpan	床上便盆
bedside commode	床边洗脸台（便桶）
bedside rails	床栏
binder	腹带、绷带
breast pump	吸奶器
bronchoscope	支气管镜
cabinet respirator	箱式呼吸器
cane (walking stick)	手杖
cannula	套管、插管
cardiac catheter	心导管
catheter	导管
cotton wool balls	棉球
crutch	拐杖
curette	刮器（耳挖、刮匙）
cystoscope	膀胱镜
defibrillator	除颤器
dialyser	渗析膜（透析器）
dialyzator	透析器
disposable collecting bag	一次性集尿袋
double current catheter	双腔导管
drainage-tube	引流管

dressing	敷料
dropper	滴管
elastic bandage	弹力绷带
electrocardiograph	心电图机
electroencephalograph	脑电图机
emesis basin	盂盆
enema can	灌肠筒
enema syringe	灌肠注射器
enemator	灌肠器
eye speculum	开睑器
female catheter	女导尿管
finger stall	指套
flexible catheter	软导管
forceps	钳子
funnel	漏斗
gastric tube	胃管
gastroscope	胃镜
gauze	纱布
glass measure cup	玻璃量杯
hemostatic forceps	止血钳
hyperbaric oxygen chamber	高压氧舱
hypodermic syringe	皮下注射器
ice bag	冰袋
incubator	保温箱
indwelling catheter	留置导尿管
intubator	插管器、喉管插入器
irrigator	冲洗器
isolation unit (set-up)	消毒室（消毒病房）
kidney basin	弯盘
mask	口罩
mattress	垫子
measuring tape	带尺
mechanical suction	机械吸吮器
medicine cup	药杯

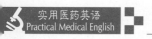

murphy's drip bulb	墨菲氏滴管
nasal speculum	鼻窥器（鼻镜）
needle	针头
negative pressure ventilator	负压呼吸机
obstetric forceps	产钳
oxygen tank	氧气筒
pacemaker	起搏器
patient pack	医院为病人提供的个人用具
percussion cannula	叩诊器
perfusion cannula	灌注套管
positive pressure ventilator	正压呼吸机
prostatic catheter	前列腺导尿管
rectal speculum	直肠窥器
rectal tube	肛管
ribbon gut	肠线
rubber-topped hemostat	带橡皮头的止血器
rubber air ring	橡皮气圈
rubber gloves	橡皮手套
rubber sheet	橡胶板
sand bag	沙袋
scalpel	手术刀
scissors	剪刀
scrotal support	阴囊托
sling	悬带
spatula (padded tongue blade)	压舌板
specimen container	取样器皿
speculum	窥器
sphygmomanometer	血压计
spirometer	肺活量计
splint	夹板
sputum suction apparatus	吸痰器
stethoscope	听诊器
stretcher	担架
sucker	吸管

suction	吸吮器
swab	拭子、药签
test tube	试管
thermometer	温度计
three-channel tube	三腔管
tourniquet	止血带
tracheal catheter	气管吸引导管
tray	托盘
ultraviolet lamp	紫外线灯
urethral speculum	尿道窥器
urinal	男用尿壶、储尿器
vaginal speculum	阴道窥器
ventilator (respirator)	呼吸机（器）
vessel clamp	止血钳、血管夹
vial	药瓶
walker	助行器
wash-out cannula	冲洗套管
wheelchair	轮椅

8) 医院部门及主要职务术语

acupuncturist	针灸师
admission office	住院处
anesthetist	麻醉师
assayer	化验师
attending physician (doctor-in-charge)	主治医师
aurist (otologist)	耳科医生
blood bank	血库
bronchoscope room	支气管镜室
cardiologist (heart specialist)	心脏专家
children's ward	儿童病房
clinical laboratory	临床化验室
consulting room	咨询室
dental department	牙科
dentist	牙医师

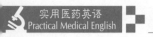

Department of Abdominal Surgery	腹外科
Department of Acupuncture	针灸科
Department of Anesthesiology	麻醉科
Department of Cardiology	心内科
Department of Cardiovascular Surgery	心血管外科
Department of Dentistry	牙科
Department of Dermatology	皮肤科
Department of Dietetics	营养科
Department of Digestive Medicine	消化科
Department of Endocrinology	内分泌科
Department of Esthetic Surgery	美容外科
Department of General Medicine	大内科
Department of General Surgery	普通外科
Department of Geriatrics	老年病科
Department of Hematology	血液科
Department of Hepatology	肝病科
Department of Internal Medicine	内科
Department of Massage	按摩科
Department of Neonatology	新生儿科
Department of Nephrology	肾内科
Department of Neuro-surgery	神经外科
Department of Neurology	神经科
Department of Obstetrics and Gynecology	妇产科
Department of Ophthalmology	眼科
Department of Orthodontics	正牙科
Department of Orthopedics	矫形外科（骨科）
Department of Otorhinolaryngology	耳鼻喉科
Department of Pathology	病理科
Department of Pediatrics	小儿科
Department of Physical Therapy	体疗科
Department of Plastic Surgery	整形外科
Department of Proctology	肛肠科
Department of Psychiatry	神经病科
Department of Radioisotope	放射性同位素科

Department of Radiology	放射科
Department of Respiratory Medicine	呼吸科
Department of Thoracic (Chest) Surgery	胸外科
Department of Traditional Chinese Medicine	中医科
dermatologist	皮肤科专家（医生）
dietitian (dietician)	营养师
diet technician	营养技术人员
director of nursing	护理部主任
disinfection room	消毒室
dispensary	药房
dispenser	药剂士
dressing room	换药室
E.C.G. room	心电图室
E.E.G. room	脑电图室
Emergency department	急诊部
Endocrinologist	内分泌专家（医生）
ENT (ear, nose, throat) Eepartment	耳鼻喉科
ENT specialist	耳鼻喉科专家（医生）
gastro-endoscopic room	胃镜室
Gastrointestinal (G.I.) Department	消化科
gastrologist	胃病专家（医生）
general office of the hospital	院部办公室
general practitioner	全科医生
general ward	普通病房
geriatrician	老年病专家（医生）
gynecologist	妇科专家（医生）
hematologist	血液科专家（医生）
hospital superintendent (director, administrator)	医院院长
In-patient Department	住院部
in-patient	住院病人
injection room	注射室
intensive Care Unit (ICU)	重症监护室
internist (physician)	内科医生
intern	实习医生

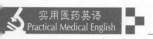

isolation ward	隔离病房
laboratory technician	化验室技术员
laryngologist	喉科医生
licensed practical nurse (LRN)	持照护士
male ward	男病房
massagist	按摩师
maternity ward	产科病房
medical director	医务主任
medical records division	病案室
medical ward	内科病房
midwife (accoucheuse)	女助产士（产科女医师）
mortuary	太平间
neonatologist	新生儿科专家（医生）
nephrologist	肾内科专家（医生）
neurologist	神经科专家（医生）
nursing assistant	助理护士（护理员）
Nursing Department	护理部
nursing education director	护理教育处长
nursing station (desk)	护理站
nursing supervisor	总护士长
observation ward	观察病房
obstetrician (accoucheur)	产科医生（男产科医生）
oculist	眼科医生
operating room	手术室
ophthalmologist	眼科专家（医生）
optical ward	眼科病房
optician	验光师
orderly	护理员（卫生员）
orthopedist	正牙专家（医生）
otolaryngologist	骨科医生
otorhinolaryngologist	耳鼻喉科专家（医生）
Out-patient Department	门诊部
out-patient	门诊病人
pathologist	病理学家

pediatrician	儿科医生
pharmaceutist (pharmacist)	制剂师
pharmacy	药房
physician's assistant	医生助理（医士）
private ward	特等病房
proctologist	肛肠科专家（医生）
psychiatrist	精神病专家（医生）
pulmonary function lab	肺功能检查室
radiologist	放射科专家
recovery room	康复室
registered nurse (RN)	注册护士
registration (registrar's office)	挂号室
resident doctor	住院医师
rhinologist	鼻科医生
stomatologist	口腔科专家（医生）
surgeon	外科医生
surgical ward	外科病房
TCM physician (doctor)	中医大夫
therapeutic room	治疗室
waiting room	候诊室
X-ray technician	X 光技术员
X-ray technologist	X 光技师

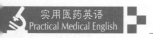
2. Commonly Used Medical Word-building Elements

a- 不，没有　　　　　anemia 贫血；apnea 无呼吸的，呼吸停止的

adeno- 腺体　　　　　adenoma 腺瘤；adenoid 腺的，淋巴组织的

-algea (-algia) 痛苦　　neuralgia 神经痛

an- 无，没有，缺乏　　analgesic 止痛的；anemia 贫血；anesthetics 麻醉剂

anti- 对抗　　　　　　antibody 抗体；antigen 抗原；antibiotics 抗生素

auto- 自己，自体　　　autograft 自体移植物；autopsy 尸检

arthr(o)- 关节　　　　arthritis 关节炎；arthralgia 关节痛

arteri- 动脉　　　　　arteriotomy 动脉切开术；arteriography 动脉 X 线摄影法

-ase 酶　　　　　　　lipase 脂肪酶；transaminase 转氨酶

audi- 听　　　　　　 auditory 听觉的；audiometer 听力计

bi- 两，双　　　　　　bipolar 双极的；bilateral 双侧的

brady- 缓慢的　　　　bradypnea 呼吸过慢；bradycardia 心动过缓

broncho- 气管　　　　bronchitis 气管炎；bronchodilator 气管扩张剂

carbo- 碳　　　　　　carbonate 碳酸盐；carbohydrate 碳水化合物

cardio- 心脏　　　　　cardiovascular 心血管的；cardialgia 胃灼痛，心痛

chemo- 化学的　　　　chemosynthesis 化学合成；chemotherapy 化疗

circum- 周围，环　　　circumcorneal 角膜周围；circumcision 包皮环切术

cranio- 颅（骨）的　　craniofacial 颅面的；craniology 头骨学，头盖学

cortico- 皮，皮质　　　corticose 皮层的；corticosteroid 皮质激素

cyst- 囊，胞膀胱　　　cystectomy 胆囊切除术；cystic 囊性的；cystitis 膀胱炎

-cyte 细胞　　　　　　erythrocyte 红细胞；thrombocyte 血小板

de- 脱离，去除，剥夺　degeneration 恶化；deoxygenate 脱氧；decongestant 解充血药

dermato- 皮肤　　　　dermatopathy 皮肤病；dermatalgia 皮痛

dys- 困难　　　　　　dyskinesia 运动障碍；dyspnea 呼吸困难；dysphagia 吞咽困难

electro- 电　　　　　 electrocardiogram 心电图；electrolyte 电解质

-emia(-hemia) 血　　　anemia 贫血；leukemia 白血病

-esthe- 感觉　　　　　esthesia 感觉，感知；anesthetics 麻醉剂

enceph(o)- 脑　　　　encephalopathy 脑病；encephalitis 脑炎

endo- 内，内部　　　　endocrine 内分泌；endotrachea 气管内；endotoxin 内毒素

epi- 在……之上　　　 epigastric 上腹部；epinephrine 肾上腺素；epicardium 心外膜

epiglott- 会厌　　　　epiglottitis 会厌炎；epiglottidectomy 会厌切除术

erythro- 红，红色　　 erythromycin 红霉素；erythematous 红斑的

-esia 疾病　　　　　　amnesia 健忘症；agennesia 无生殖力

-esis 疾病　　　　　　　tyremesis 吐乳症；diuresis 利尿

ex- 自……出来，排出　　excrete 排泄；expectorant 化痰的，化痰剂

exo- 外部的　　　　　　exotoxin 外毒素；exocrine 外分泌

febri- 发烧　　　　　　febricide 退热剂；febrile 热性的

fibr(o)- 纤维　　　　　fibrocyte 纤维细胞；fibrosis 纤维化，纤维变性

-fus(e)- 合并，注入　　infusion 灌输，输液；transfusion 输液，输血

gastr(o)- 胃　　　　　gastrointestinal 胃肠道的；gastritis 胃炎

gene 基因　　　　　　generation 产生；genetic 遗传的

genitor- 生殖，生殖器　genitourinary 泌尿生殖的

-gia 疼痛　　　　　　neuralgia 神经痛；arthralgia 关节痛

globule 球　　　　　globulin 球蛋白；globulimeter 血细胞计算器，血球计算器

hemo- 血，血液　　　hemoglobin 血红蛋白；hemophilia 血友病；hemorrhage 出血

histo- 组织　　　　　histocyte 组织细胞；histology 组织学

hydrate 水化物　　　hydratase 水和酶；dehydrate 脱水

hyper- 高，过多　　　hypertension 高血压；hyperinflation 过度膨胀；hypercardia 心肥大

hypo- 低于，不足　　hypotrophy 不足生长；hypotension 低血压；hypotonic 张力下降

-ia 疾病　　　　　　dyspepsia 消化不良；aphasia 失语症；diphtheria 咽喉炎

-iasis 疾病　　　　　elephantiasis 象皮病；siriasis 中暑

idio- 特殊的，自己的　idiopathy 特发病，自发病；idioparasite 自体寄生物

-igo 疾病　　　　　　vertigo 晕眩；porrigo 头癣

-ism 疾病　　　　　　deaf-mutism 聋哑症；nicotinism 尼古丁中毒症

-itis 炎症　　　　　　meningitis 脑膜炎；bronchiolitis 细支气管炎；laryngitis 喉炎

intra- 内，内部　　　intracellular 细胞内的；intracranial 颅内的

-itis 炎　　　　　　gastritis 胃炎；hepatitis 肝炎；nephritis 肾炎

-kine- 运动　　　　　kinesimeter 运动测量计；akinesia 运动不能

lacer- 撕裂　　　　　lacerant 令人痛苦的；laceration 伤口，裂口

lateral 侧边　　　　unilateral 单侧的；trilateral 三边的

leuk-(leuc-) 白　　leucocyte 白细胞；leukemia 白血病

litho 结石，石　　　lithotomy 结石切除术；lithotrity 碎石术

lymph- 淋巴　　　　lymphadenopathy 淋巴腺疾病；lymphangiitis 淋巴管炎

-ma 斑，瘤　　　　myoma 肌瘤；sarcoma 肉瘤，恶性毒瘤

mal- 坏，不良　　　malignant 恶性的；malabsorption(营养)吸收不良；malformation 畸形

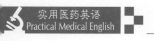

mening(o)- 脑膜　　　　　meningitis 脑膜炎；meningioma 脑（脊）膜瘤

-meter 测量　　　　　　　audiometer 听力计；kinesimeter 运动测量计

muco- 黏膜　　　　　　　mucosa 黏膜；mucocutaneous 黏膜皮肤的

multi- 多　　　　　　　　multisystem 多系统的；multiple 多样的，多重的

nat(us)- 出生　　　　　　prenatal 产前的，出生前的；natality 出生率，出生

neutro- 中　　　　　　　neutrocyte 中性粒细胞；neutropenia 中性粒细胞减少症

neo- 新　　　　　　　　　neomycin 新霉素；neonate 新生儿；neonatal 新生期的

nephro- 肾　　　　　　　nephrocyte 肾细胞；nephrotoxicity 肾毒性；nephrosis 肾病

non- 非，不，无　　　　　nonabsorbable 不能被吸收的；noninfectious 非传染的

-ology 学　　　　　　　　biology 生物学；psychology 心理学

-oma 疾病　　　　　　　　neuroma 神经病；xanthoma 黄色瘤

-ostomy 切开术，造瘘术　　tracheostomy 气管切开术；colostomy 结肠造瘘术

orch(o)- 睾丸　　　　　　orchotomy：睾丸切开术；orchitis 睾丸炎

or(o)- 口　　　　　　　　oral 口头的

-osis 疾病　　　　　　　　tuberculosis 结核病；necrosis 坏死

ot(o)- 耳　　　　　　　　otitis media 中耳炎；otitis 耳炎；otophone 助听器；otolith 耳石

-ox(ygen)- 氧气　　　　　hypoxia 低氧血症；oxygenic 氧的，含氧的

para- 副，侧面　　　　　　parablast 副胚层；paramyxovirus 副黏病毒

-path(y)- 疾病　　　　　　neuropathy 神经病；nephropathy 肾病；pathogenetic 发病的，致病的

-penia 血细胞减少　　　　thrombocytopenia 血小板减少症；neutropenia 中性粒细胞减少症

per- 穿透　　　　　　　　perfusion 灌注；perforate 打孔

pharyng(o)- 咽　　　　　pharyngitis 咽炎；pharyngalgia 咽痛

-phil- 嗜　　　　　　　　neutrophil 嗜中性白细胞；hemophilia 血友病

-phago- 吞咽，吞噬　　　　phagocyte 吞噬细胞；dysphagia 吞咽困难

photo- 光，相片　　　　　photophobia 畏光；photoactive 光（激）活的，光敏的

-phobia 恐惧症　　　　　　acrophobia 恐高症；basophobia 步行恐惧症

pneumo- 肺，气　　　　　pneumonia 肺炎；pneumococcus 肺炎球菌

-pnea 气体，呼吸　　　　　apnea 呼吸停止；dyspnea 呼吸困难

poly- 多　　　　　　　　　polyacid 多元酸；polyphagia 多食症

pro- 居前，领先　　　　　proenzyme 酶原；prodromal 前驱的，有前驱症状的

psycho- 心理，精神　　　　psychopathy 心理病态；psychology 心理学；psychosexual 性心理

pulmo- 肺　　　　　　　　pulmometer 肺量计；pulmonary 肺的

reticul(o)- 网状的　　　　reticular 网状组织；reticuloendothelial 网状内皮的

rheumat(o)- 风湿 rheumatoid 类风湿的；rheumatic 风湿性的 rheumatic fever 风湿热

-rrhea 大量流出 diarrhea 腹泻；steatorrhea 脂肪泻

soma- 体 somatic 肉体的；somasthenia 躯体无力

-spir(ate)- 通气 respiration 呼吸；inspire 吸气

steato- 脂肪 steatoma 脂肪瘤；steatorrhea 脂肪泻

steno- 狭窄 stenocephaly 头狭窄，小头；stenosis 狭窄

strepto- 链状 streptomycin 链霉素；streptococcus 链球菌

sub- 下，亚，次 subcutis 皮下组织；submaxillary 下颌的

syn- 共同，联合 synkinesia 协同性运动，辅助运动；syncytial 合胞病毒的

-thermo- 体温，热度 thermometer 体温计；hyperthermia 高热

tracheo- 气管 tracheotomy 气管切开术；tracheobronchial 气管支气管的

tachy- 快，迅速 tachypnea 呼吸过快；tachycardia 心动过速

-tension 压力，张力 hypertension 高血压；hypotension 低血压

thrombo- 血小板，血栓 thrombosis 血栓症；thrombocytopenia 血小板减少症

trans- 转移 transfusion 输血；transfer 转移，转让，传递

-tomy 切 anatomy 解剖学；appendectomy 阑尾切除术

-tonic- 强身的（药） cardiotonic 强心的，强心剂；tonicity 强壮，肌肉弹性

umbil- 脐 umbilectomy 脐切除术；umbilical cord 脐带

-uria 尿 oliguria 少尿；hematuria 血尿

vaso- 血管，输精管 vasodilation 血管扩张；vasoactive 血管活性的

vascul- 血管 vasculitis 脉管炎，血管炎；vascularity 血管分布

xanth(o)- 黄 xanthopathy 黄变症；xanthaematin 血黄素

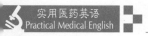

3. Medical Abbreviations

a.a.	of each, *from Latin, ana* 每
Ab	antibody 抗体
ABD or abd	abdomen 腹部
ABG	arterial blood gases 动脉血气
ABX	antibiotics 抗生素
a.c.	before food, *from Latin, ante cibum* 饭前
ADH	antidiuretic hormone 抑制尿分泌激素
ADL	activities of daily living 日常活动
ad lib	as desired *from Latin, ad libitum* 按需
adm	admission 入院，接收住院
ADR	adverse drug reaction 药物不良反应
Ag	antigen 抗原
a.h.	every other hour, *from Latin, alternis horis* 每隔一小时
AI	artificial insemination 人工授精
AIDS	Acquired Immune Deficiency Syndrome 获得性免疫缺陷综合征
ALS	advanced life support 高级生命支持
altern. d.	every other day, *from Latin, alterno die* 每隔一天
AMA	advanced maternal age (35 years or older) 高产龄
AMI	acute myocardial infarction 急性心肌梗塞
ANS	autonomic nervous system 自主神经系统
AP	antero-posterior 前后位
a.p.	before dinner, *from Latin, ante prandium* 饭前
aq.	water, *from Latin, aqua* 水
aq. bull.	boiling water, *from Latin, aqua bulliens* 开水
aq. calid.	warm or hot water, *from Latin, aqua calida* 热水
aq. dist.	distilled water, *from Latin, aqua distillata* 蒸馏水
aq. gel.	cold water, *from Latin, aqua gelida* 冷水
ARDS	acute respiratory distress syndrome 急性呼吸道窘迫综合征
ARF	acute renal failure 急性肾衰竭
aur.	ear, *from Latin, auris* 耳
aur. dextro.	to right ear, *from Latin, auris dextrae* 右耳
aur. laev	to left ear, *from Latin, auris laevae* 左耳
Ba	barium 钡

BCX	blood culture 血液培养
b.i.d.	twice daily, *from Latin, bis in die* 每日两次
BGL	blood glucose level 血糖水平
bl.cult	blood culture 血液培养
BLS	basic life support 基础生命支持
BM(bm)	bowel movement 排大便
BMR	basal metabolic rate 基础代谢率
BMT	bone marrow transplantation 骨髓移植
BP	blood pressure 血压
BP	bipolar disorder 双相障碍
BPD	borderline personality disorder 临界人格紊乱
BPH	benign prostatic hyperplasia 良性前列腺增生
BS	blood sugar 血糖
BSL	blood sugar level 血糖水平
BUN	blood urea nitrogen 血尿素氮
Bx	biopsy 活检
C	centigrade 摄氏
CABG	coronary artery bypass graft 冠状动脉搭桥术
CAD	coronary artery disease 冠状动脉疾病
CAG	coronary artery graft 冠状动脉移植术
CA	carcinoma, cancer 肿瘤
Ca	calcium 钙
CAH	congenital adrenal hyperplasia 先天性肾上腺增生
CAT	computed axial tomography 计算机轴向断层扫描
cath	catheter 导管
CBC	complete blood count 全血细胞计数
CC	cubic centimeter, or chief complaint 立方厘米，主诉
CHD	coronary heart disease 冠心病
CHF	congestive heart failure 充血性心力衰竭
CK	creatine kinase 肌氨酸激酶
CKD	chronic kidney disease 慢性肾脏疾病
CLL	chronic lymphocytic leukemia 慢性淋巴细胞白血病
CML	chronic myelogenous leukemia 慢性淋骨髓性白血病
CNS	central nervous system 中枢神经系统

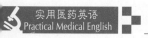

COAD	chronic obstructive airways disease 慢性阻塞性呼吸道疾病
COLD	chronic obstructive lung disease 慢性阻塞性肺部疾病
COPD	chronic obstructive pulmonary disease 慢性阻塞性肺部疾病
CO	cardiac output 心脏输出量
CO, C/O	complains of … 主诉
CO	carbon monoxide 一氧化碳
CO_2	carbon dioxide 二氧化碳
CP	chest pain 胸痛
CPR	cardiopulmonary resuscitation 心肺复苏
CRF	chronic renal failure 慢性肾脏衰竭
CS	caesarean section 剖腹产
CSF	cerebrospinal fluid 脑脊液
CT	computed tomography 计算机断层扫描术
CVA	cerebrovascular accident 脑血管意外
CVC	central venous catheter 中心静脉插管
CVD	cardiovascular disease 脑血管疾病
CVP	central venous pressure 中心静脉压
Cx	microbiological culture 微生物培养
CXR	chest X-ray 胸部透视
DBP	diastolic blood pressure 舒张压
DDD	daily defined doses 每日规定剂量
DDx	differential diagnosis 鉴别诊断
DIC	disseminated intravascular coagulation 扩散性血管内凝血
DJD	degenerative joint disease 退行性关节疾病
DM	diabetes mellitus 糖尿病
DNA	deoxyribonucleic acid 脱氧核糖核酸
DOA	dead on arrival 到达时已死
DOB	date of birth 出生日期
Dx	diagnosis 诊断
ECG	electrocardiogram 心电图
ED	emergency department 急诊科
EDD	estimated date of delivery 预产期
EDD	estimated date of discharge 预计出院日期
EEG	electroencephalogram 脑电图

EKG	electrocardiogram 心电图
ELISA	enzyme-linked immunosorbent assay 酶联接免疫吸附剂测定
ENT	ear, nose and throat (otolaryngology) 耳鼻喉
ER	emergency room 急诊室
F	farenheit 华氏
FBC	full blood count 全血计数
FBG	fasting blood glucose 空腹血糖
FBS	fasting blood sugar 空腹血糖
FHR	fetal heart rate 胎儿心率
FHx	family history 家族史
ft.	foot or feet 英尺
Fx	fracture of a bone 骨折
g	gram 克
GA	general anaesthesia 全身麻醉
gal.	gallon 加仑
GH	growth hormone 生长激素
GI	gastrointestinal 胃肠道的
GU	genitourinary 泌尿生殖的
H/A	headache 头痛
HAV	hepatitis A virus 甲型肝炎病毒
Hb	hemoglobin 血色素
HBV	hepatitis B virus 乙型肝炎病毒
HCT	hematocrit 血球容积计
HCV	hepatitis C virus 丙型肝炎病毒
HDL	high density lipoprotein 高密度脂蛋白
HDL-C	high density lipoprotein cholesterol 高密度脂蛋白胆固醇
HDV	hepatitis D virus 丁型肝炎病毒
HEV	hepatitis E virus 戊型肝炎病毒
HGB	hemoglobin 血色素
HIV	human immunodeficiency virus 人类免疫缺陷病毒
HLA	human leukocyte antigens 人类白细胞抗原
HPI	history of present illness 目前疾病史
HR	heart rate 心率
H.S.	at bedtime, *from Latin, hora somni* 睡觉时；hour of sleep 睡眠

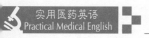

HT	hypertension 高血压
HTN	hypertension 高血压
I131	radioactive iodine 放射性碘
IA	intra-arterial 动脉内的
IC	intracardiac 心脏内的
ICD	international classification of diseases 国际疾病分类
ICP	intracranial pressure 颅内压
ICU	intensive care unit 重症监护病房
I&D	incision and drainage 切割和引流
IDA	iron deficiency anemia 缺铁性贫血
IDL	intermediate density lipoprotein 中等密度脂蛋白
Ig	immunoglobulin 免疫球蛋白
IGT	impaired glucose tolerance 糖耐量受损
i.m.	intramuscular 肌肉内
IMI	intramuscular injection 肌内注射
INF	interferon 干扰素
I&O	inputs and outputs 输入和输出
IOP	intraocular pressure 眼内压
IQ	intelligence quotient 智力商数
IUCD	intrauterine contraceptive device 子宫内避孕用具
i.v.	intravenous 静脉内
IVDU	intravenous drug user 静脉注射吸毒者
IVP	intravenous pyelogram 静脉注射肾盂造影
K	potassium *from German, kalium* 钾
Kcal	kilocalorie 卡
Kg	kilogram 千克
L	leukocytes 白细胞
LDH	lactate dehydrogenase 乳酸盐脱氢酶
LDL	low density lipoprotein 低密度脂蛋白
LDL-C	low density lipoprotein cholesterol 低密度脂蛋白胆固醇
Leu	leukocytes 白细胞
LFT	liver function test 肝功能测试
LMP	last menstrual period 末次月经
Lp	lipoprotein 脂蛋白

LP	lumbar puncture 腰椎穿刺
LPL	lipoprotein lipase 脂蛋白脂肪酶
LUL	left upper lobe 左上叶
Ly	lymphocytes 淋巴细胞
MCHC	mean cell hemoglobin concentration 红细胞平均血红蛋白浓度
MCH	mean cell hemoglobin 红细胞平均血红蛋白
MCV	mean cell volume 平均细胞容积
Mg	magnesium 镁
MI	myocardial infarction 心肌梗塞
Mod	moderate 中等的
Mo	monocyte 单核细胞
MPV	mean platelet volume 平均血小板容积
MRA	magnetic resonance angiography 磁共振血管造影
MRI	magnetic resonance imaging 磁共振成像
Na	sodium *from German, natrium* 钠
NA	nursing assistant 护理员
NAD	no abnormality detected 未见异常
NBM	nothing by mouth 禁食
NE	norepinephrine 去甲肾上腺素
Neo	neoplasm 肿瘤
Nil	none 没有
NPO	nothing by mouth, *from Latin, nil per os* 禁食
NREM	non-rapid eye movement 非快速动眼期
n.s.	not significant 不明显
NS	normal saline 生理盐水
NTG	nitroglycerin 硝化甘油
N&V	nausea & vomiting 恶心和呕吐
NVD	nausea, vomiting & diarrhea 恶心、呕吐和腹泻
NVD	normal vaginal delivery 正常阴道分娩
O_2	oxygen 氧
OA	osteoarthritis 骨关节炎
OB-GYN	obstetrics and gynecology 产科与妇科
OD	right eye, *from Latin, oculus dexter* 右眼
OD	overdose 剂量过多

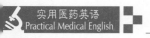

od	every day, usually regarded as once daily 每日，每日一次
OGTT	oral glucose tolerance test 口服葡萄糖耐量实验
om	every morning, *from Latin, omni mane* 每日早晨
on	every night, *from Latin, omni nocte* 每晚
OP	outpatient department 门诊部
OS	left eye, *from Latin, oculus sinister* 左眼
OS	orthopedic surgery 整形外科
OTC	over-the-counter drug 非处方药
OU	both eyes, *from Latin, oculi uterque* 双眼
p	(p with a bar over it) after, *from Latin, post* 在……之后
PA	pulmonary artery 肺动脉
PAH	pulmonary arterial hypertension 肺动脉高压
p.c.	after food, *from Latin, post cibum* 餐后
PE	pulmonary embolism 肺栓塞
PE	physical examination 体格检查
PLT	platelets 血小板
p.o.	by mouth (orally), *from Latin, per os* 口服
postop	postoperative 手术后
PPH	post partum haemorrhage 产后出血
PPH	primary pulmonary hypertension 原发性肺动脉高压
p.r.	per rectum (rectal) examination 直肠检查
preop	preoperative 术前
p.r.n	as necessary, *from Latin, pro re nata* 必要时
Pt.	patient 患者
PT	physical therapy 体疗
PVD	peripheral vascular disease 外周血管疾病
PVR	pulmonary vascular resistance 肺血管阻力
Px	prognosis 预后
q	each, every, *from Latin, quaque* 每
q.a.d.	every other day, *from Latin, quaque altera die* 每隔一天
q.AM	every AM, *from Latin, quaque ante meridiem* 每天早晨
q.d.	each day, *from Latin, quaque die* 每天
q.d.s.	four times each day, *from Latin, quater die sumendus* 每日四次
q.h.	each hour, *from Latin, quaque hora* 每小时

q.h.s.	every bedtime, *from Latin, quaque hora somni* 每晚就寝时
q.i.d.	four times each day, *from Latin, quater in die* 每日四次
q.m.t.	every month 每月
q.w.k.	weekly 每周
q.o.d	every other day 每隔一天
RA	refractory anaemia 难治性贫血
RA	rheumatoid arthritis 风湿性关节炎
RAI	radioactive iodine 放射性碘
RBC	red blood cell count 红细胞计数
REM	rapid eye movement 快速眼动期
RFT	renal function test 肾脏功能测试
RhF	rheumatoid factor 风湿因子
RLQ	right lower quadrant 右下腹部
ROM	range of motion 环绕关节的运动，全关节运动图
RR	respiratory rate 呼吸率
RUQ	right upper quadrant 右上腹部
RV	right ventricle 右心室
RVF	right ventricular failure 右心室衰竭
RVSP	right ventricular systolic pressure 右心室收缩压
Rx	medical prescription or prescription drug 处方药
SARS	severe acute respiratory syndrome 严重急性呼吸道综合征
SBE	subacute bacterial endocarditis 亚急性细菌心内膜炎
SBP	systolic blood pressure 收缩压
SBP	spontaneous bacterial peritonitis 自发性细菌腹膜炎
SC	subcutaneous, *from Latin, subcutis* 皮下
SHx	surgical history 手术史
SOB	shortness of breath 气促
SOS	save our souls 急救
STD	sexually transmitted disease 性传播疾病
STI	soft tissue injury 软组织损伤
SVI	systemic viral infection 系统性病毒感染
TB	tuberculosis 肺结核
TF(T/F)	transfer 转院，转科
THR	total hip replacement 全髋关节置换术

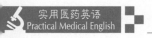

TIA	transient ischemic attack 短暂性脑缺血发作
t.i.d.	three times a day, *from Latin, ter in die* 每日三次
TKR	total knee replacement 全膝关节置换
TLC	total lung capacity 肺总容量
TOP	termination of pregnancy 妊娠终止
TPN	total parenteral nutrition 全胃肠道外营养
TT	thrombin time 凝血酶时间
TTE	transthoracic echocardiogram 经胸廓心回波图
Tu	tumour 肿瘤
TUR	transurethral resection 经尿道切除术
Tx	treatment 治疗
UBT	urea breath test 尿素呼气实验
URTI	upper respiratory tract infection 上呼吸道感染
US	ultrasound 超声
USG	ultrasonography 超声波检查法
USS	ultrasound scan 超声波扫描
UTI	urinary tract infection 尿道感染
VA	visual acuity 视觉敏度
VC	vital capacity 肺活量
VD	vaginal delivery 产道分娩
VE	vaginal examination 阴道检查
VF	ventricular fibrillation 心室纤维性颤动
VLDL	very low density lipoprotein 极低密度脂蛋白
WBC	white blood cell count 白细胞计数
WDWN	well developed, well nourished 发育良好，营养良好

4. Scripts of Conversation B

Unit One

Conversation B

Receiving a Patient

(Episode One)

Doctor: Good morning. I am Doctor Sterling. How can I help you?

Patient: Good morning, Doctor. I am Emily. I have had a fever and sore throat since yesterday.

Doctor: Oh, did you take your temperature?

Patient: Yes, I did. The highest temperature was 39.8℃ at 11 p.m. last night. I took one pill of aspirin and felt much better.

Doctor: Any other symptoms?

Patient: I have a runny nose and headache, too.

Doctor: Ok, let me take your temperature first. Please keep this thermometer under your armpit for 5 minutes. Open your mouth and say "Ah", please. Your tonsils and larynx are red and swollen. Your temperature is 38.5° C. Your breathing sounds are normal and there is no problem with your lungs. You'd better take the blood test, ok? This paper is for the lab test.

Patient: Sure. I really hope I can get better as soon as possible. See you later.

Key Words & Phrases

sore /sɔː/ *adj.* 疼痛的

sore throat 咽喉痛

aspirin /'æsp(ə)rɪn/ *n.* 阿司匹林

thermometer /θə'mɒmɪtə/ *n.* 温度计，体温表

tonsil /'tɒns(ə)l/ *n.* 扁桃体

larynx /'lærɪŋks/ *n.* 咽喉

blood test 血液检查

(Episode Two)

(30 minutes later, the patient comes back.)

Patient: Excuse me, doctor. Here's the result of my blood test.

Doctor: Ok. The blood routine shows that your WBC is 12,000/mm^3, N80%, L20%. It indicates that you have an upper respiratory tract infection. Are you allergic to any drugs or foods?

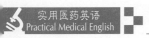

Patient: No. I don't think so.

Doctor: I'll prescribe Amoxicillin for you. It's an oral medicine. Take 2 tablets 3 times a day around the clock. You can take aspirin if fever persists. You'd better take vitamin C—2 tablets 3 times a day, too. And drink a lot of liquids and have plenty of rest.

Patient: How long should I take the medicine?

Doctor: Take it for 5 days, and come back for a follow-up check-up. Don't hesitate to call me if you have any problems.

Patient: Thank you so much. I really appreciate your help.

Key Words & Phrases

blood routine 血常规

WBC (white blood cell) 白细胞

upper respiratory tract infection 上呼吸道感染

allergic /əˈlɜːdʒɪk/ *adj.* 过敏的

Amoxicillin /əˌmɒksəˈsilin/ *n.* 阿莫西林

follow-up /ˈfɒləʊʌp/ *n.* （对患者的）随访

Unit Two

Conversation B

Consulting a Doctor
(Episode One)

Doctor: Hi, I am Doctor Susan. How can I help you?

Patient: Hi, doctor. I am Mary. Would you please take a look at my lab result?

Doctor: Sure. Take a seat, please.

Patient: Thank you. This is the blood result of my kidney function, and the other is the liver function.

Doctor: I see. I'd like to know your medical history first. Have you had any problems with your kidney or liver?

Patient: Yes. I was told I had IgA nephropathy five years ago because both my uric acid and creatinine were too high. My urine has been tea-colored for almost five years.

Doctor: Did you have a biopsy?

Patient: No. The doctor suggested the biopsy but I am really afraid of that. So they haven't been able to diagnose the IgA until now.

Doctor: What kind of symptoms do you have now?

Patient: Oh, I have had gout for a week, and my left foot is still painful and swollen.

Key Words & Phrases

    lab result 实验室检查结果

    kidney function 肾功能

    IgA (immunoglobulin A) nephropathy 免疫球蛋白 A 肾病

    urine acid 尿酸

    creatinine /krɪˈætɪniːn/ *n.* 肌酐

    biopsy /ˈbaɪɒpsɪ/ *n.* （活组织）切片检查

    gout /gaʊt/ *n.* 痛风

(Episode Two)

Doctor: May I take a look at your foot? Ah, I see. Are you taking any medication?

Patient: Yes. I am taking a pain killer for my gout these days. But I don't remember the name of the medication.

Doctor: Your present lab results are good, the urine acid and creatinine are normal. You'd better avoid the painkillers since they affect kidney function.

Patient: Good. Your instructions are really helpful. Do I need any other medications for my gout?

Doctor: You could try some Chinese traditional herbs, such as notoginseng, to enhance your blood circulation.

Patient: Oh, really? I haven't heard that before. But I have heard that Chinese traditional medicine does cure some sicknesses. I'd like to try.

Doctor: Ok, you can buy some from the drug store.

Patient: Thank you so much. I really appreciate your instructions. Have a good day!

Doctor: You're welcome. Have a good day.

Key Words & Phrases

    pain killer 止痛药物

    herb /hɜːb/ *n.* 中草药

    notoginseng /nəʊˈtɒdʒɪnseŋ/ *n.* 三七

    enhance /ɪnˈhɑːns/ *v.* 提高，增强

    blood circulation 血液循环

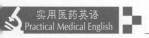

Unit Three

Conversation B

Admitting a Patient

(Episode One)

Nurse: Good morning, Mrs. Wilson. I am the nurse of the GI Department. My name is Emily. I'll be admitting you to the ward today.

Patient: Good morning, Emily. What should I do now?

Nurse: Would you please come with me to the nurses' office so I can finish the paperwork first?

Patient: Sure. May I sit down?

Nurse: Yes, of course. Please sit down and make yourself comfortable, OK? Can you tell me your full name and your date of birth?

Patient: My full name is Rose Wilson. And I was born on Nov. 15th, 1968.

Nurse: Can you tell me why you are here today?

Patient: Well, um. I've had a duodenal ulcer for about five years. My stools have been black for the past two days. I feel weak, too. My occult blood test is positive, so my doctor suggested I come here.

Key Words & Phrases

admit /əd'mɪt/ *v.* 许可进入

admit a patient 收病人入院

GI Department 消化科

GI (gastrointestinal /ˌgæstrəʊɪn'testɪn(ə)l/) *adj.* 胃肠的

duodenal /ˌdjuːəʊ'diːnəl/ *adj.* 十二指肠的

ulcer /ˌʌlsə(r)/ *n.* 溃疡

stool /stuːl/ *n.* 大便

(Episode Two)

Nurse: Ok. Would you please give me your past results, such as the barium X-rays and gastrointestinal endoscopy? We need to make a copy and put it into your chart.

Patient: Sure. I'll give them to you later.

Nurse: By the way, I'd like to know your past medical history. Have you had any serious illnesses in the past except the duodenal ulcer?

Patient: No. I think my duodenal ulcer came from too much pressure in my job. I am busy with my work every day so I can't take good care of myself.

Nurse: Mm, that's reasonable. I'll take the BP for you now. I'd like you to sit a little closer to this desk and roll up your sleeve. Ok，it's one ten over 70, that's good. I'd also like to take your pulse rate.

Patient: Is my pulse too fast？ I always feel palpitations these days.

Nurse: Mm, a little bit fast. It's one fifteen. And please put this thermometer under your tongue. You can take it out when you hear the beep. Ok, it's 37.0 ℃. Thank you very much for your cooperation, Mrs. Wilson. Now please follow me, and I will show you around the ward.

Key Words & Phrases

barium /'beərɪəm/ *n.* 钡

barium X-rays X 线钡餐检查

gastrointestinal endoscopy 胃肠道内镜

endoscopy /en'dɔskəpi/ *n.* 内视镜检查法

chart /tʃɑːt/ *n.* 病历

BP (blood pressure) 血压

pulse rate 脉率

palpitation /pælpi'teiʃ(ə)n/ *n.* 心悸

Unit Four

Conversation B

In the Nurses' Office

(Episode One)

Doctor: Hello. Mary, are you looking after Mr. John today？

Nurse: Yes. Any questions？

Doctor: Oh, can we take a few minutes to talk about his situation？

Nurse: Sure. Have a seat, please.

Doctor: Thank you. He was back from the OR an hour ago and there are a lot of orders for him. Let's make sure they are clear.

Nurse: Ok. Let me see. Blood pressure, pulse rate, breathing rate every 30 minutes, temperature every 4 hours. And monitor the GCS every 4 hours.

Doctor: And also monitor his I & O, OK？

Nurse: Sure. How about his fluids？

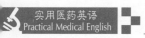
Doctor：Now his potassium levels are very low according to his blood result. Would you please give him a liter of Normal Saline with 20 millimoles of KCL?

Nurse: Sure. Please fill out the patient's chart first.

Key Words & Phrases

      OR (Operation Room) *n.* 手术室

      order /'ɔ:də/ *n.* 医嘱

      GCS (Glasgow Coma Scale) *n.* 格拉斯哥昏迷评分量表

      I&O (intake and output) *n.* 出入量

      potassium /pə'tæsiəm/ *n.* 钾

      liter /'li:tə/ *n.* 升

      millimole [mɪlɪ'mɒl] *n.* 毫摩尔

      Normal Saline *n.* 生理盐水

(Episode Two)

Doctor: No problem. Thanks for your reminder. The Normal Saline with 20 millimoles of KCL should be given over 4 hours, ok?

Nurse: I see. Any other fluids？

Doctor: Yes. I will prescribe some antibiotics for him. I'd prefer you to run them through a secondary line (第二条静脉通路).

Nurse: Ok. May I run them through the cannula?

Doctor: Right. Make sure the cannula is still working because we didn't use it yesterday. And I want to give him some nutrients with the fluids. These nutrients are sticky, so you can't run them through the cannula in case of blockage.

Nurse: I understand.

Doctor: Furthermore，start him on some oxygen at 2 liters per minute for 3 hours because his oxygen saturation is 90. We also need to monitor his oxygen saturation, OK?

Nurse: Of course. Don't forget to fill out all these orders, doctor.

Key Words & Phrase

      antibiotic /ˌæntɪbaɪ'ɒtɪk/ *n.* 抗生素

      cannula /'kænjʊlə/ *n.* 导管，套管

      nutrient /'nju:trɪənt/ *n.* 营养物，营养品

      blockage /'blɒkɪdʒ/ *n.* 堵塞

saturation /ˌsætʃəˈreɪʃ(ə)n/ *n.* 饱和度

oxygen saturation 血氧饱和度

Unit Five

Conversation B

Administering Medications

(Episode One)

Nurse: Hi, Janice, Good to see you again.

Patient: Thank you and me too. You look so nice today.

Nurse: How are you doing today?

Patient: Not good, I have a headache and feel dizzy today. My blood pressure was one eighty over one ten (180/110) this morning. That's really high, isn't it?

Nurse: Oh, I see. That's the reason why Dr. Peter prescribed two new medications for you. One is Metoprolol, to lower your BP. And another is Lasix, a diuretic.

Patient: Oh, I can't remember the names. Would you please repeat them?

Nurse: Sure, and I'll tell more about them. Metoprolol is in the green box, and I already wrote down the instructions for you. You take these two pills twice a day, that's 8 a.m. before your breakfast and 8 p.m. before your bedtime. Got it?

Patient: Mm, but I have a very poor memory. Instructions on the box are good for me.

Key Words

dizzy /ˈdɪzi/ *adj.* 头晕眼花的，眩晕的

Metoprolol /metɒpˈrɒlɒl/ *n.* 美托洛尔

Lasix /ˈleɪsɪks/ *n.* 速尿（呋喃苯胺酸制剂的商品名）

diuretic /ˌdaɪjuˈretɪk/ *n.* 利尿剂

(Episode Two)

Nurse： OK, let's continue. You have to put this medicine in a cool place because it would be melt at 45 ℃. Another one, Lasix, is in the white box. It's a diuretic (water pill) that prevents your body from absorbing too much salt, allowing the salt to be eliminated through the urine instead. This medication is also used to treat hypertension.

Patient: Does that mean I will pass more urine after I take this medication?

Nurse: Yes, absolutely. The frequency and amount of your urine will be increased. But don't worry, that's the normal effect of the medication. Please let us know if you

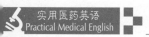
aren't comfortable or have any problems, OK?

Patient: Thank you. Any other instructions?

Nurse: Oh, by the way, you'd better eat a low-cholesterol, low-fat, low-sodium diet with more dietary fiber. That means that you'd better eat more fresh vegetables and fruits, less salt and meat. That's good for both your hypertension and heart.

Patient: That's really very hard for me. Anyway, I'll try my best to follow your guidance. You are a great nurse.

Key Words

urine /ˈjʊərɪn/ *n.* 尿

cholesterol /kəˈlestərɒl/ *n.* 胆固醇

sodium /ˈsəʊdɪəm/ *n.* 钠

dietary /ˈdaɪət(ə)rɪ/ *adj.* 与饮食有关的，饮食的

fiber /ˈfaɪbə/ *n.* 纤维

Unit Six

Conversation B

Preoperative Nursing
(Episode One)

Nurse: Morning, Mrs. Peter. I am Cathy. Did you sleep well last night?

Patient: Morning, Cathy. I was a little nervous about the surgery, so I didn't sleep that well.

Nurse: Yes, it's hard for everyone at this point. Do you have any questions about the surgery?

Patient: Mm, I signed the consent form two days ago, and I saw the risks of the operation in the form, such as the complications from the anesthesia, the bleeding, and even death. I am a little afraid of these things.

Nurse: *(smiles and touches the patient's hand)* I understand it's not easy for you. Actually the consent form tells us all kinds of possibilities during the surgery, but these risks are very small and not likely to happen to you. It's just standard hospital procedure.

Patient: I see. I hope my surgery is successful, especially my child is only five years old.

Nurse: *(smiles)*It will be fine. You should trust the doctors. And you have been on a low-residue diet for 3 days, right?

Patient: Yes. May I eat today?

Nurse：Yes, but only clear fluids for today. Then you'll start NPO after midnight.

Key Words & Phrases

preoperative /prɪˈɒpərətɪv/ *adj.* 手术前的

consent form 知情同意书

anaesthesia /ˌænəsˈθiːzɪə/ *n.* 麻醉

low-residue diet 少渣饮食

NPO (nothing per mouth) 禁食

(Episode Two)

Patient: Does that mean I won't be able to eat or drink anything after midnight?

Nurse: No, you won't. And you will be given an enema tonight around 8 p.m.

Patient: For what? Is it painful?

Nurse: The enema causes you to have a bowel movement and then lower the risk of contamination from the bowel contents. It won't be painful; I am sure you can handle it.

Patient: Ok. If I have to, I will.

Nurse: There are two more things before the surgery. Tomorrow morning you'll be given a nasogastric tube to keep the stomach empty. You'll keep the tube for a few days for gastric decompression. It will also lower the pressure of the incision.

Patient: Oh, my goodness! I hope that's all.

Nurse: It's good for you to know all the details of your procedure. The other tube you'll have is an indwelling catheter, which can be taken out when you can void by yourself. I'll take care of you before and after the operation tomorrow. You'll be just fine.

Key Words & Phrases

enema /ˈenəmə/ *n.* 灌肠

bowel /ˈbaʊəl/ *n.* 肠

contamination /kənˌtæmɪˈneɪʃən/ *n.* 污染

nasogastric tube 鼻胃管

decompression /diːkəmˈpreʃ(ə)n/ *n.* 减压

incision /ɪnˈsɪʒ(ə)n/ *n.* 切口

indwelling catheter 留置尿管

void /vɒɪd/ *v.* 排泄

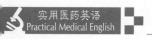

Unit Seven

Conversation B

Postoperative Nursing Discussion

(Episode One)

Head Nurse: Hello, everyone. Let's start with Mrs. John. Mrs. John is a 40-year-old American lady and was admitted last Friday. From her biopsy she was diagnosed with rectum cancer 6 months ago in our hospital. A colostomy was performed on her at 10 a.m. yesterday. She is fully awake and recovered from the procedure. We are going to talk about her nursing implementations, especially the stoma care after the surgery.

Nurse 1: Mm, I examined her yesterday after she came back from the OR. I feel that she's doing well. Her vital signs are good, except for a slight fever. But that's normal after the surgery. The stoma is swollen, but the blood circulation around the stoma is good.

Nurse 2: Yes, we need to pay close attention to the stoma.

Head Nurse: What kind of stoma is normal, post-op?

Nurse 1: Stoma is initially edematous and shrinks over the next 4 to 6 weeks. A normal stoma is moist and reddish pink. I think Mrs. John's is a standard.

Key Words & Phrases

rectum cancer 直肠癌

colostomy /kə'lɒstəmɪ/ *n.* 结肠造口术

nursing implementations 护理措施

stoma /'stəʊmə/ *n.* 造口

post op 手术后

edematous /ɪ'diːmətəs/ *adj.* 水肿的

shrink /ʃrɪŋk/ *v.* 收缩

(Episode Two)

Head Nurse: Any other signs? How about the skin?

Nurse 2: The skin is intact and free of irritation. And we should continue to monitor the condition of the stoma.

Head Nurse: Good. It sounds that you know everything of the observation. Let's move on. How about the application of the pouching system? We should talk about the steps of the pouching system.

Nurse 1: The first step is to wash our hands and apply clean gloves. And then place a towel across the patient's lower abdomen to protect bed linen. Remove the used pouch and skin barrier gently.

Head Nurse: Mary, do you want to follow? You must have some ideas.

Nurse 2: Mm, the skin around the stoma should be cleaned with warm water using a washcloth. Measure the stoma before cutting an opening on skin barrier. After that, the protective backing will be removed. Then apply pouch over the stoma.

Head Nurse: Perfect! By the way, don't forget to close the end of the pouch if it is open. You guys did a wonderful job with the discussion. Thank you. Have a good day!

Nurses: You too.

Key Words & Phrases

intact /ɪn'tækt/ *adj.* 完整无缺的；未经触动的；未受损伤的

irritation /ɪrɪ'teɪʃn/ *n.* 刺激

pouching system　造瘘袋

skin barrier　皮肤黏着物

washcloth /'wɒʃklɒθ/ *n.* 擦洗布

protective backing　*n.* 保护层

Unit Eight

Conversation B

Enema

(Episode One)

Nurse: Hi, Mrs. John. How are you today?

Patient: Not bad. How are you?

Nurse: Good. I hear you've been constipated for a few days.

Patient: Yes. I haven't had a bowel movement at least four days so my abdomen feels distended and painful. I took some medicine but it doesn't work.

Nurse: That must be uncomfortable. Dr. Peter ordered an enema for you.

Patient: Oh, what is enema? Will it hurt?

Nurse: An enema is a tube of liquid inserted into the rectum through the anus to help your bowel movements. It won't hurt. I am sure you can handle it.

Patient: Ok, I hope so. What should I do now?

Nurse: You should go to the bathroom first. I'll go to prepare the stuff and come back later.

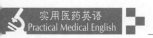

Key Words

distend /dɪ'stend/ *v.* 膨胀，肿胀

rectum /'rektəm/ *n.* 直肠

anus /'eɪnəs/ *n.* 肛门

(Episode Two)

(The nurse comes back a few minutes later.)

Nurse: Mrs. John. Are you ready?

Patient: Yes.

Nurse: Ok, would you please show me your identification bracelet? Ok, thanks. Now take off your pants to the knees and lie on your left side. Good, bend your knees, please.

Patient: Could you let me know when you start?

Nurse: Sure. Now take deep breaths. Good. Now there we go. How are you feeling now?

Patient: Is it done? I feel very uncomfortable.

Nurse: Please keep this position for 5 to 10 minutes and then you can go to the bathroom. Please ring the bell if you need me.

Patient: Thank you so much. I appreciate your help.

Key Phrases

identification bracelet 腕带识别卡

lie on one's left side 左侧卧位

bend one's knees 屈膝

take a deep breath 深呼吸

Unit Nine

Conversation B

Health Education
(Episode One)

Nurse: Hi, Mrs. Peter. How are you today?

Patient: Good. How are you?

Nurse: Very good. Thank you. I'd like to talk about your diabetes management before your discharge.

Patient: Oh, thanks. I am really worrying about the complications of the diabetes after I go back home.

Nurse: I understand it's not easy for you to manage it now, so we need to educate you first.

Patient: I think so.

Nurse: OK, let's start. There are two types of diabetes, type 1 and type 2. Do you know what type you have?

Patient: Type 2. It's also called non-insulin-dependent diabetes. And the doctor suggested that I take the insulin injections.

Nurse: Good. Can you tell me how many units have been prescribed for you?

Patient: 4 units of regular insulin. But I am not sure.

Key Words & Phrases

complication /kɒmplɪˈkeɪʃ(ə)n/ *n.* 并发症

non-insulin-dependent diabetes 非胰岛素依赖型糖尿病

insulin /ˈɪnsjʊlɪn/ *n.* 胰岛素

regular insulin 常规胰岛素

(Episode Two)

Nurse: That's correct. 4 units of insulin mark 0.1 millimoles for the 1ml syringe. Remember to inject the insulin 30 minutes before your meal. It'll be more convenient for you if you can afford the insulin pen. Most diabetics use insulin pen because its prefilled devices are disposable and easy for them.

Patient: Oh, I've heard that before. I hope I can.

Nurse: Ok. You need to control your weight and nutrition, too. Some regular physical activities are good for you but do not try to exercise too much at one time. Always bring some snacks with you to prevent hypoglycemia.

Patient: Ok, I see. But it's more difficult for me to control the nutrition because I am always hungry.

Nurse: I understand. But you must control your food according to doctors' orders in case of hyperglycemia.

Patient: My husband is always talking about that, too. I will try.

Nurse: Good. Here is a pocket booklet of diabetes management. Bring it with you.

Key Words

syringe /sɪˈrɪndʒ/ *n.* 注射器

disposable /dɪˈspəʊzəb(ə)l/ *adj.* 一次性的

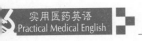

hypoglycemia /ˌhaɪpəuɡlaɪˈsiːmɪə/ *n.* 低血糖

hyperglycemia /ˌhaɪpəɡlaɪˈsiːmɪə/ *n.* 高血糖

Unit Ten

Conversation B

Intravenous Therapy

(Episode One)

Nurse: Morning, Miss Susan. I am Mary. I will be looking after you today.

Patient: Morning, Mary. Pleased to meet you. How does my urine culture look? I can't handle the pain anymore. Today I have to go to the bathroom more often.

Nurse: Your urine culture indicated you have a urinary tract infection. And Doctor Wilson prescribed intravenous antibiotics according to your sensitivity test.

Patient: You mean you will give me an IV right now?

Nurse: Yes, if you are ready.

Patient: Ok. Do I need to take the skin test first?

Nurse: No need. But you can go to the bathroom first and I will come back later.

Patient: Sure. See you later.

Key Word & Phrases

urine culture 尿培养

urinary tract infection 尿路感染

IV /ˌaɪˈviː/ 静脉输液

skin test 皮试

(Episode Two)

(A few minutes later, the nurse comes back.)

Nurse: Susan, are you ready?

Patient: Yes. Will it hurt?

Nurse: Mm, just a little bit. Not much. May I check your identification bracelet first?

Patient: Sure, here you are.

Nurse: Ok, thanks. Please lie down and make yourself comfortable. Hold your hand for a minute. Good. Now relax your hand. There we go.

Patient: Oh, that wasn't bad. You did a good job.

Nurse: Thank you. You'd better not to change the dripping rate. Keep your hand in whenever you move.

Patient: Alright.

Nurse: Please ring the call bell if you need help.

Key Phrases

dripping rate 滴速

call bell 呼叫铃

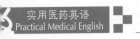

5. Text Translation

Unit 1

Text A

化学即生活

你知道"每种生物为了生存都依赖于化学"这个事实吗？当你了解到所有动植物的生命材料以及发生在动植物身上的所有变化从本质上讲都是化学变化时，你就会对这一事实有更加清楚的理解。事实上，化学是一门牵涉到所有材料的构成及材料所经历的变化的科学。

人体是一个化工厂。食物作为向人体提供能量和构建组织所必不可少的物质，必须通过消化系统的化学过程才能溶解，被消化系统溶解的食物只能通过人体细胞内的化学过程才能向人体提供能量和构建组织。人体腺体所产生的物质被输送到人体的各个部位。这些物质可以决定你的智力是否正常以及你是胖还是瘦这样一些重要特征。此外，使你知冷知热，为你提供嗅觉并使你的感觉和思考的神经系统也依赖化学反应。

植物的生命与化学的密切关系也显而易见。除非发生某些化学变化，否则植物不能生存。植物内的化学变化使它吸收空气中的二氧化碳并将其用于生产养分及繁殖细胞。在这一过程进行时，所有动物生命所必需的氧气就与空气联系在了一起。通过这些化学变化，人类及所有的动物生命所需的食物及氧气就得到了保证。因此，植物使得生命成为可能。

每天人们为了生存而使用的所有普通产品都是化学产品。医生为了治病所开的处方药，你为了预防感染所使用的抗生素，你为了牙齿清洁所使用的牙膏，你为了保持身体洁净所使用的肥皂，都是化学实验室试验出的产品。

通过对化学的了解和应用，工业已经提供了许多使人们生活更加愉快和方便的产品，尼龙、合金和塑料就是其中几个例子。

Text B

人体结构与功能

解剖学涉及人体结构与功能。通过学习解剖学，人们会理解每个器官系统的基本概念和原理，以及他们如何保持人体的动态平衡。

人是世界上最复杂的生物。在我们的身体中，无数独特的精细部件以一种有组织的方式，一起在为整个生命的存在而运行。组成人体的无数细小结构主要分为四种。

细胞是维持和繁殖生命的最简单的生命物质单位。人体由无数细胞组成，最开始是单个的受精细胞。人体有不同种类的细胞，如白细胞、红细胞和血小板。

组织是比细胞更复杂一些的单位。组织是由许多相似细胞，以及细胞间不同数量和种类的无生命细胞间物质组成的结构。

器官是具有特殊功能的不同组织结合起来形成的东西。例如，胃是由肌组织、结缔组织、上皮组织和神经组织构成。肌组织和结缔组织形成胃壁，上皮组织和结缔组织形成胃的内层，神经组织遍布胃壁和内层。

系统是人体组成部分中最复杂的。系统由不同数量和种类的器官组成，执行人体复杂的功能。人体主要有十种系统：骨骼系统、肌肉系统、神经系统、内分泌系统、心血管系统、淋巴系统、呼吸系统、消化系统、泌尿系统和生殖系统。

机体功能包括身体系统的生理和心理功能。生存是机体之要务。生存依赖于机体的动态平衡，即内环境相对稳定状态的保持与恢复。

身体的动态平衡取决于身体不断从事各种活动。身体的主要活动或功能包括对人体环境变化做出反应、在环境和细胞间交换物质、代谢食物及整合身体的不同活动。

身体的许多功能逐年变化。一般说来，身体在幼年和老年时期的功能最差。在儿童时期，身体功能日趋有效和高效。在成熟后和老年期则相反。在成人早期，身体功能的效力和效率最高。

Text C

生命过程

生命的基本过程包括组织、新陈代谢、反应性、运动和繁殖。对人类而言，生命过程还要包括生长、分化、呼吸、消化和排泄。所有这些过程相互关联，一起维持着个体生命。疾病和死亡代表着对生命平衡过程的破坏。下面是对生命过程的简要介绍。

组织　人体所有层次的组织安排都存在分工。人体的每一个组成部分都有自己特定的任务，并与其他部分合作。单个细胞如果失去完整性或组织性，也会死去。

新陈代谢　新陈代谢包括身体内发生的所有化学反应。新陈代谢的一个阶段叫作分解代谢。分解代谢时，复杂的物质被分解成更简单的组成材料，释放能量。

反应性　反应性也叫兴奋性，即对内外环境变化的觉察并对该变化做出反应，也可以说是对刺激的觉察和反应。

运动　身体内有许多类型的运动。在细胞层面，分子在运动。血液在身体各处运动。每次呼吸，横膈膜会运动。

繁殖　生命通过生物体的繁殖代代相传。从广义上讲，繁殖还指为了生长以及替换或修复老细胞而形成新细胞。

生长　生长指由于细胞数量增加或个体细胞增大而形成的体积增大。机体要生长，那么合成代谢的速度一定要高于分解代谢的速度。

分化　分化是一种发育过程，在这个过程中，未分化细胞转化成具有独特结构和功能特征的专门化细胞。通过分化，细胞发育成组织和器官。

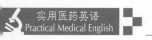
呼吸　呼吸指在细胞和外部环境间氧气和二氧化碳交换的所有过程。

消化　消化指个体摄取的复杂物质被分解成可被血液吸收和机体利用的简单分子的过程。

排泄　排泄指从身体中排除消化和新陈代谢过程中所产生的废物的过程。排泄会排除身体不能利用的副产物，其中包括很多有毒的和与生命不相容的物质。

除了上述十种生命过程之外，生命还依赖环境中的某些物理因素，包括水、氧气、营养物、热量和压力等。

Unit 2

Text A

美食人生

我们的身体是非常复杂的。我们只能在一定的体温范围内维持生命并且发挥身体的正常功能。正如大家所知，一个成人的正常体温是 37℃。身体必须维持这个温度而不管外部温度如何变化。为了做到这一点，身体必须产生足够的热量和能量，使其能够运行重要的生物过程，如肌肉运动、消化、呼吸、血液循环等。为了获得这种能量，每个人都要吃饭或摄取食物。在经历了数百道复杂的化学过程之后，我们所吃的食物就变成了人体发挥正常功能的必需物质。食物在构建新组织，修复坏死细胞方面也是必不可少的。

在一生中，你大概要消耗掉 50 吨食物。食物所含的最主要成分是碳水化合物、脂肪和油类、蛋白质、矿物质和维生素。尽管水并不产生能量，但它对人体正常功能的发挥是必不可少的。任何程度的水的缺失都将扰乱人体内各种液体的正常浓度并且使许多器官不能正常地发挥功能。

碳水化合物是我们饮食的一部分。碳水化合物是含有碳、氢和氧的有机化合物。在碳水化合物里，氢和氧的比例与在水中的比例相同，即两个氢原子对应一个氧原子。最普通的碳水化合物是糖分和淀粉。

脂肪和油类也是饮食的组成部分，这些营养成分包括碳、氢、氧。它们以不同的比例出现。动植物的脂肪和油类是脂的混合物，在正常情况下，是液体的被称为油类；是固体的被称为脂肪。它们是人体内的第二类能量来源。

蛋白质是很复杂的氮化合物。碳水化合物和脂肪是人体活动的主要能源，但它们不是人体组织的主要构成成分。例如肌肉组织只含有极少量的碳水化合物和少量的脂肪。肌肉及动植物细胞的原生质的主要成分通常是被称为蛋白质的化合物。由于氮的存在，蛋白质与碳水化合物和脂肪得以区别开来，因为蛋白质含有大约 16% 的氮。

人体内的原生质占了人体重量的 4% 以上。动物组织含有许多种无机化合物，它们是从食物中获取的。这些食物就变成了人体不同组织的一部分。

Text B

普通感冒

普通感冒，亦称上呼吸道感染，是一种由诸多不同类型病毒所致的传染性疾病。由于导致感冒的病毒数量众多，新的感冒病毒不断出现，人体不能对所有感冒病毒都产生抵抗力，因此，感冒易频发和复发。

普通感冒的症状有鼻塞、流鼻涕、咽喉疼痛、声音嘶哑、咳嗽，还有可能包括发烧和头痛。许多感冒患者感到疲倦和疼痛。这些症状一般会持续三到十天。

无论患者是否服药，感冒通常会在几天到数周时间里好转。但是，感冒病毒会引起其他感染侵袭人体，这些感染包括鼻窦感染、耳部感染和支气管炎。即使在感冒消失后，哮喘、慢性支气管炎或肺气肿患者的症状也可能在数周内加剧。

普通感冒大多通过手部接触传染。例如，感冒患者流鼻涕，用手接触鼻子，然后接触其他人，其他人就会被病毒感染。此外，人们还可能被钢笔、书籍、咖啡杯子等物体上的感冒病毒感染。尽管常识表明咳嗽和打喷嚏会传播感冒病毒，但事实上这些并非传播感冒病毒的常见方式。

一般说来，抗生素药物治疗感冒并无疗效。抗生素药物只是对细菌导致的疾病有疗效，而感冒通常由病毒所致。抗生素药物不仅没有帮助，反而可能导致致命的过敏性反应。还有，滥用抗生素药物已经导致几种常见细菌对抗生素药物产生了耐药性。由于上述及其他原因，限制抗生素药物的使用显得十分重要。有时，感冒病毒之后会出现细菌感染。普通感冒产生的细菌性并发症可用抗生素药物治疗。

有几种缓解感冒症状的疗法。解充血药和鼻用喷剂有助于缓解感冒症状。心脏病患者、高血压控制不良者和患有其他疾病的人在使用这些药物之前应该与医生联系。而且，鼻用喷剂非处方药的使用不应超过三天，因为鼻部可能产生赖药性，中止使用这些药物可能会产生更严重的鼻塞。

Text C

肺炎

肺炎是由各种病因导致的肺部感染，包括细菌、病毒、真菌、寄生虫感染，以及肺部的化学或物理损伤。在抗生素药物被发现以前，有三分之一的肺炎患者都会死于感染。今天，肺炎仍旧是老年人和慢性疾病末期患者的一个主要死因。

肺炎的典型症状有咳嗽、胸痛、发热和呼吸困难。传染性肺炎患者通常出现伴有绿痰或黄痰的咳嗽症状，以及出现伴随寒战的高热。气短也常见。肺炎患者可能咯血、头痛、出汗或觉得湿冷。其他可能出现的症状有食欲不振、皮肤发青、恶心、呕吐、情绪波动以及关节疼痛或肌肉疼痛。

医务工作者依据病人症状和其体格检查结果来诊断肺炎。胸部透视、血液检查和痰培

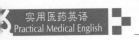

养也有助于诊断。有放射设备的医院和诊所诊断肺炎时常用胸部透视。为鉴别肺炎和其他疾病，偶尔需用胸部 CT 扫描或其他检查。

大多数肺炎病例不需要住院治疗。一般情况下，口服抗生素药物、卧床休息、补充体液和家人照料便足以完全解决问题。然而，呼吸困难、有其他疾病或年老的肺炎患者可能需要进一步治疗。如果症状加剧，在家治疗后病情没有改善，或有并发症发生，病人则必须住院接受治疗。

人们常使用抗生素药物治疗细菌性肺炎。相反，抗生素药物对病毒性肺炎并无用处。是否选用抗生素药物取决于肺炎的性质。理想的肺炎治疗应建立在针对具体致病微生物及其对抗生素的敏感性的基础上。

因肺炎呼吸困难者需要额外吸氧，重病患者需重症监护治疗，包括插管和人工呼吸。

有时肺炎会导致其他并发症。细菌性肺炎比病毒性肺炎更易导致并发症。最常见的并发症有呼吸和循环衰竭、胸膜渗液、肺水肿、肺脓肿等。

护理肺炎病人时的护理措施和职责包括按处方给氧、给药并监测其效果，对生命体征的监测，监听肺鸣音，观察肺水肿和病人气促的感觉。如果病人卧床不能移动，则有必要每两小时给病人翻一次身，鼓励病人咳嗽和深呼吸。

Unit 3

Text A

心肺复苏术

如果你在电视里看过有关医院的场景，你也许看见过心肺复苏术。心肺复苏术也被简称为 CPR，它能挽救生命。下面让我们来看看它是怎样发挥作用的吧。

什么是 CPR？

Cardio 表示 "有关心脏的"；Pulmonary 表示 "有关肺的"；Resuscitation 是一个医学名词，意思是复苏，即挽救生命。CPR 常常能救活一个呼吸已停止，心脏也许停跳的病人。

实施 CPR 的人，即施救者，主要遵循三个步骤，即 C—A—B：

C：胸部按压；

A：检查呼吸；

B：人工呼吸。

胸部按压

施救者在做 CPR 时应使用双手，即一只手按压在另一只手上，对病人胸部进行多次按压，以压出骤停心脏中的血液。

这一系列被称为胸部按压的动作有助于把含有氧气的血液压送到人体各重要器官，尤其是至关重要的大脑。长时间大脑缺氧会导致一个人死亡。

在每一次按压动作的间隙间，应把病人的双手举起来，让胸廓复位。此举会让血液重新流回心脏。这样的话，在等待医疗紧急救助和医辅人员来接送病人到医院之前，施救者会通过持续的救助让血液和氧气流向病人的大脑和身体各部分，从而不让其死亡。

检查呼吸

在完成 30 次按压后，施救者应检查病人是否还有呼吸。

人工呼吸

如病人已无呼吸，应给与两次救助呼吸。这就是人工呼吸。为了实施人工呼吸，施救者应将自己的嘴放在病人的嘴上吹气，以迫使空气进入病人肺部。（为避免实际接触，救助者最好使用特殊的口罩）。人工呼吸有助于把氧气输入已停止呼吸的病人的肺部。在完成两次人工呼吸后，施救者应继续对病人实施胸部按压。

何时该实施 CPR？

CPR（胸部按压、检查呼吸和人工呼吸）应被用于抢救一个呼吸停止、心脏骤停的病人。当你突遇紧急情况发生，有人病得很严重的时候，你应尽最大努力保持镇静。首先，你应轻拍病人的肩部，同时提问："你还好吗？"以观察病人有无反应。在病人已无反应，你又具备 CPR 资格的情况下，可开始实施 CPR。如你独自一人，又无法实施 CPR，则应大声呼救或拨打紧急求救电话 120。

谁应掌握 CPR？

特定人群应该知道如何实施 CPR。包括医生、护士、医辅人员、急诊医技人员在内的医学专业人员务必掌握 CPR。救生员、儿童工作者、学校教练、训练员等人群也必须掌握 CPR 技能。家里有心脏病及其他病症患者的人也应学会实施 CPR。

Text B

严重急性呼吸道综合征

严重急性呼吸道综合征 (SARS) 是由 SARS 冠状病毒 (SARS-CoV) 导致的一种人类呼吸道疾病。该病在 2002 年 11 月到 2003 年 7 月曾广泛流行过一次。世界卫生组织 2004 年 4 月 21 日公布的报告显示，在此期间全球共有 8 090 例已知感染病例，774 例死亡（死亡率 9.6%）。

2002 年 11 月 1 日到 2003 年 7 月 31 日的 SARS 病例

国家或地区	病例	死亡	死亡率 (%)
中国大陆	5 328	349	6.6
中国香港	1 755	299	17
加拿大	251	43	17
中国台湾	346	37	11
新加坡	238	33	14

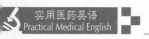
续表

国家或地区	病例	死亡	死亡率 (%)
越南	63	5	8
美国	27	0	0
菲律宾	14	2	14
德国	9	0	0
蒙古	9	0	0
泰国	9	2	22
法国	7	1	14
马来西亚	5	2	40
瑞典	5	0	0
意大利	4	0	0
英国	4	0	0
印度	3	0	0
韩国	3	0	0
印度尼西亚	2	0	0
南非	1	1	100
中国澳门	1	0	0
科威特、爱尔兰、罗马尼亚、俄罗斯、西班牙、瑞士	每国 1 例	0	0
总计	8 090	774	9.6

（本表内容是根据世界卫生组织公布的资料整理的。）

SARS 的最初症状类似流感，可能有发热、肌痛、精神萎靡、胃肠道症状、咳嗽、咽喉肿痛和其他非典型症状。所有病人唯一共有症状是 38℃以上的发热。病人后来可能会呼吸短促。一般说来，病人在接触病毒 2 ～ 10 日后出现症状，但也有人在 13 日左右才出现症状，在大多数情况下 2 ～ 3 天内出现症状。

SARS 的胸部透视结果不定。最初的胸部透视可能是清晰的。白细胞和血小板计数通常很低。

由于 SARS 是病毒性疾病，抗生素药物没有疗效。到目前为止治疗 SARS 很大程度上是用退热剂，必要时补充氧气，进行通气支持。必须隔离 SARS 疑似病人。

最初传言类固醇和抗病毒药病毒唑对 SARS 有疗效，但并无公开发表数据证实这种疗法。许多临床医生现在怀疑病毒唑有害。研究人员目前正在测试所有已知用于治疗 AIDS、肝炎、流感和其他疾病的抗病毒药物对 SARS 冠状病毒的疗效。

有迹象表明，SARS 导致的一些较严重损害是由机体本身免疫系统对病毒的过度反应所致。使用类固醇和其他免疫调解药物治疗发病较急的 SARS 病人可能有一些好处。这方面的研究工作正在进行。

Text C

禽流感

禽流感也称 H5N1。这种疾病与猪流感、犬流感、马流感和人类流感相似，都是由已适应某特定物种的不同株系流感病毒所致。

禽类像人类一样会染上流感。禽流感病毒感染的对象包括鸡、鸭、其他家禽和野鸟等禽类。然而，禽流感也会对人类的健康产生威胁。1997 年在中国香港出现了第一例直接感染人类的禽流感病毒，H5N1。此后，禽流感病毒扩散到了亚洲、非洲和欧洲的许多国家。

人类感染禽流感病毒虽然少见，但是导致鸟类感染的病毒会变化或变异，然后更容易使人类感染。这样会导致禽流感大范围流行，或在全世界暴发。

在禽流感病毒暴发期间，与受到感染的禽类接触过的人群会生病。吃没有煮熟的家禽或接触已感染人群也可能使人生病。禽流感病毒会使人重病甚至会致人死亡。目前还没有出现能预防该疾病的疫苗。

禽流感病毒在鸟类中自然存在。全世界的野鸟的肠道中存在这种病毒，但它们一般不会因此生病。然而，禽流感病毒在家禽中传染性很强，会使鸡、鸭、火鸡等家禽患病死亡。

感染了禽流感病毒的鸟类的唾液、鼻涕和粪便中包含病毒。易感鸟类在接触此类含病毒的分泌物或排泄物时，或接触被此类分泌物或排泄物污染的物体表面时，就会感染禽流感病毒。家禽感染禽流感病毒的途径有直接接触已感染水禽或家禽，或接触被禽流感病毒污染的表面（如尘土或鸟笼）或物质（如水或饲料）。

人类禽流感的症状有典型的人类流感样症状（如发热、咳嗽、咽喉肿痛和肌肉疼痛），眼睛感染，肺炎，严重呼吸道疾病（例如急性呼吸道窘迫），以及其他严重威胁生命的并发症。禽流感的症状取决于导致感染的病毒类型。

已有实验室研究表明，一些处方药在治疗人类禽流感感染方面应该有效。但是，禽流感病毒会对这些药物产生耐药性，因此这些药物并非总是有效。人们需要更多的研究来证实这些药物的有效性。

Unit 4

Text A

中国传统医药

中草药是世界上伟大的草药系统之一，其连绵不绝的传承可以追溯到公元前 3 世纪。

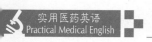

在其历史中，为适应不断变化的临床疾病，中草药在不断发展，并且通过对其各方面应用进行的研究得到了支撑。这个过程随着现代医疗诊断技术和医学知识的发展而持续到了今天。

因为其系统性的方法和临床的有效性，中医几百年来对东方医学的理论和实践都有着巨大的影响，近年来在西方也得到了广泛而迅速的发展。在中国，草药一直是健康保健的重要组成部分，并且在国家医院里和西药一起被采用。

中医包括了所有出现在东南亚且源于中国的东方传统医学。中医医生可能按照某种源于日本、越南或韩国的传统医学工作。中医是一套完整的医学系统，能治疗范围广泛的疾病。中医包括草药疗法、针灸、食疗、呼吸与运动的训练（太极和气功）。其中的某些方法可以用于疾病的治疗。

中草药和中医的其他部分均以阴阳概念为基础。其目的就是要理解阴阳二者间可能存在的基本平衡与协调，理解人的气息或生命力可能耗损或阻断的方式，并用这些理论治疗疾病。临床策略以反映身体失衡的体征和症状的模式为基础。

然而，这种传统医学总的来说强调生活方式的调节，这样做就是为了预防疾病的发生。中医认为健康并不只是不生病，它特有的潜能就是保持和增强人体机能以获得健康和快乐。

大量研究表明传统植物疗法的应用和已知的植物成分的药理活动常常是一致的。然而，草药不同于以药学为基础的药物。第一，因为植物成分的复杂性远比以孤立的活动成分为基础的药物更为平衡，并大大降低了引发副作用的可能性。第二，因药方一般是多种草药的组合，里面各种不同成分相互平衡，共同作用，提高了疗效与安全性。第三，中草药主要寻求修正体内失衡而不只是治疗病症，治疗措施是要激励身体的自愈。

Text B

脑出血

脑出血是脑内血管破裂导致的颅内出血。

脑出血可发生在大脑的任何部位。血液可能会积聚在脑组织本身，或是在大脑和脑膜覆盖的空间之间。出血可能只发生在一个脑半球，但也有可能发生在其他脑组织。脑出血可能由脑外伤、脑肿瘤或血管畸形所致。除此之外，高血压也常导致脑出血。出血会刺激脑组织，造成肿胀（脑水肿）。出血也可能聚集形成血肿。水肿或血肿都将增加脑组织的压力并迅速毁掉脑组织。

出血的位置和受影响的脑组织的数量会导致不同的症状。症状通常发生在人们活动时，发生得迅速且无预兆。它会引起头痛、恶心、呕吐，引起意识、视觉、知觉、运动水平的变化，还会造成吞咽、读写、语言表达和理解的困难，以及导致协调和平衡能力的丧失。

脑出血是一种严重的疾病，需要马上医治。它可能会很快危及生命。治疗要根据出血的位置、原因和程度而定。可能需要手术，尤其是小脑出血。通过手术也可以修补或除去引起出血的组织。使用的药物可能包括止痛剂，可以消除肿胀的皮质激素类药物和利尿剂，以及可控制癫痫发作的抗癫痫类药物。还可使用血液、血液制品和静脉注射液来补充所损失的血液和水分。另外根据个体状况的差异和病情的发展也可采用其他的治疗方法。

病人的恢复程度取决于血肿的大小和水肿的数量。病人也许会完全康复，也许会永久地丧失某些大脑功能。即使得到及时医治，病人也可能会死亡，甚至很快死亡。药物治疗、外科手术或其他治疗都可能产生严重副作用。

治疗和控制潜在的疾病可以降低发生脑出血的风险。高血压应进行治疗，若无医生告知，切勿停药。动脉瘤通常可以在导致脑出血之前得到治疗。

Text C

糖尿病

糖尿病是一系列以高血糖为特征的代谢性疾病。高血糖则是由胰岛素分泌缺陷或其生物功能受损，或二者兼有引起的。

糖尿病可能导致失明、肾衰竭和神经损伤。以上病症是由于微小血管受损，即微血管病变引起的。糖尿病也是加快动脉硬化和变窄（动脉粥样硬化）的重要因素，从而导致中风、冠心病和其他大血管病变。

未经治疗的糖尿病早期症状与升高的血糖水平和葡萄糖在尿液中的流失有关。尿液中葡萄糖过多可造成尿量增加，并导致脱水。脱水引起的口渴会导致摄水量增多。胰岛素不能正常发挥作用会影响蛋白质、脂肪和碳水化合物的代谢。胰岛素是促进合成代谢的一种激素，能促进脂肪和蛋白质的贮存。糖尿病患者虽然食欲增大，但胰岛素的相对或绝对不足最终会导致其体重减轻。一些未经治疗的糖尿病患者也会出现疲劳、恶心和呕吐。糖尿病患者易发生膀胱、皮肤和会阴部感染。血糖波动可导致视力模糊。血糖太高可导致嗜睡和昏迷。

糖尿病主要有两种，即1型和2型。1型糖尿病也称为胰岛素依赖型糖尿病，或青少年发病型糖尿病。在1型糖尿病中，胰腺受到自身免疫系统的攻击而不能产生胰岛素。2型糖尿病也称为非胰岛素依赖型糖尿病，或成人发病型糖尿病。2型糖尿病的患者仍可以产生胰岛素，但相对而言不能满足身体的需要，尤其是在面对胰岛素抵抗时。

积极加强对1型和2型糖尿病患者体内高血糖的控制，可以减少肾病、神经病变和视网膜病变的并发症，并有可能减少大血管病变的发生和恶化。积极的控制和强化治疗可使患者的空腹血糖水平达到70～120毫克每分升；饭后血糖水平低于160毫克每分升。

治疗糖尿病的目标是使血糖水平接近正常，达到尽可能安全的水平。此外，由于糖尿病有可能极大地增加患者患心脏病的危险，积极控制血压和胆固醇的预防性措施也是目前糖尿病治疗的重要部分。

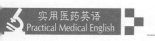

Unit 5

Text A

CT 检查

在 CT 扫描前 4 小时你可能被要求禁食。做腹部或盆腔 CT 前，肠道需要事先被处理为不透明。这一步可通过在扫描前饮用钡剂或碘剂来实现，通常在扫描前 10 分钟或 1 ～ 2 小时，有时 12 小时前完成。通常不需要其他的特殊准备。但是，扫描盆腔之前，有时可能需要服用一点灌肠剂。对于一些妇产科的扫描而言，可能要求使用卫生棉条。

在 CT 扫描室内，你要躺在一张检查台上。检查台徐徐地移动，穿过 CT 机中央的孔。在扫描过程中，你可能需要接受静脉注射碘剂或造影剂。这些物质通过血液循环，会突出许多器官并且使异常部位更加明显。

碘剂可通过肾脏迅速排出体外。身体有热感，口中有金属味是常有感觉。这种感觉很快就会过去。对碘剂产生恶心、呕吐和过敏反应则很少见。肾功能不良的人不能接受这种碘剂注射，服用盐酸二甲双胍（降血糖药）的糖尿病患者应在扫描前先抽血检查肾功。

碘剂通常在肘部或腕部被注射进静脉。在扫描之前可由医生手动注射，也可在扫描过程中由注射泵完成。在扫描期间，X 射线管围绕你旋转。它隐藏在机器里，所以你看不见。在扫描期间，你可能被要求屏住呼吸。虽然完成整个过程可能需要长达 30 分钟，包括准备时间、打印和检查图像的时间，但常规扫描仅需 20 秒到 2 分钟。扫描时间的长短应根据扫描的类型而定。

图像打印出来后，放射医师将对其进行研究并且给出报告。诊断医生通常在 24 小时内拿到报告。但若是遇到急诊，可立刻拿到报告。

Text B

消化性溃疡

消化性溃疡是胃或者十二指肠内壁出现的一些疮口，通常是由幽门螺旋杆菌引起的。胃产生盐酸和酶，其中酶包括用来消化食物的胃蛋白酶。黏膜层覆盖在胃内壁上，它起到保护胃免遭胃酸侵蚀的作用。前列腺素也可以保护内膜。当这些保护物不起作用的时候，盐酸和酶就会逐步破坏内膜，形成的疮口就叫作溃疡。幽门螺旋杆菌是一种尿素酶产生的细菌，它能破坏胃产生的黏膜。虽然幽门螺旋杆菌的感染出现在很多病例中，但并不是所有的溃疡都是由它引起的。如果长期使用非甾类化合物，如阿司匹林、萘普生、布洛芬，也会引起消化性溃疡。

十二指肠溃疡的常见症状是持续的腹部隐痛，常发生在饭后数小时或者夜间，并伴随食物的中和而减轻。体重减轻、腹胀、恶心一般不会被用作判断依据。急剧、突然、持续的胃痛，带血或者黑色大便，呕吐或带血呕吐等临床表现常被用作判断依据。

由幽门螺旋杆菌引起的消化性溃疡的实验室诊断有各种方式和样本类型。最普遍的实验室检查是幽门螺旋杆菌抗体的血样测试。幽门螺旋杆菌抗体的出现意味着你在过去的某个时候被感染过。大便的取样能够收集幽门螺旋杆菌抗原，这种检查可能不适合那些在大便中有血的个例。呼吸测试也能查出幽门螺旋杆菌酶的活动。一些侵入式的检查也能够检查胃溃疡，这些方法包括在 X 射线引导下的胃和十二指肠的内窥镜检查，也就是将末端装有微型摄像机的一根细小导管从口腔经食管插入十二指肠进行检查。

消化性溃疡不是一种致命的疾病，但是如果溃疡穿破了胃或者十二指肠（穿孔），破坏了血管（引起出血），或者有块状物停留在胃里（障碍物），那就会很严重。通常的处理方式是通过抗生素化合物来杀死细菌或者减少胃酸的产生。

Text C

急性肾衰

急性肾衰是一种肾的重要功能（即从血液中排除过多体液和废物的功能）的突然消失。若肾丧失了过滤功能，你的身体就会出现体液失衡和废物聚集的情况。

在就医的肾病人群中，急性肾衰的症状最常见。特殊人群甚至需要重症护理。急性肾衰常发生在复杂的手术后，或者严重受伤等导致的对肾的血液供应中断时。

肾功能的衰竭也会随着时间的推移逐步发展，早期的临床表现及症状并不明显。这种情况通常被认为是慢性肾衰，高血压和糖尿病是引起慢性肾衰的主要原因。

与慢性肾衰不同，急性肾衰是很严重的，通常需要精心的护理。尽管如此，急性肾衰是可逆的。如果你身体很健康，几周内就可以自动恢复。如果急性肾衰发生在慢性病程中，如心脏病的发作、阵痛、急性感染，后果就会很严重。

急性肾衰的临床表现和症状包括：

尿量减少；

体液潴留（可导致大腿、踝部或脚部水肿）；

气促；

疲劳；

代谢紊乱；

重症患者可出现谵妄或昏迷；

心包炎（囊状膜的发炎包围心脏）引起的胸痛。

很多人没有足够重视早期症状，或者只是更担心导致突发肾衰的潜在问题。

肾是两个蚕豆形的器官，有人的拳头那么大，位于脊柱两侧，紧贴腹后壁，居腹膜后方。它们分泌尿液，排出代谢废物、毒物和药物。血液首先通过身体大动脉的分支——肾动脉进入肾，然后从肾动脉流向每个肾单位。

每一个肾脏主要由约 100 万个具有相同结构与机能的肾单位和少量结缔组织所组成，其间有大量血管和神经纤维。

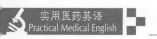

新陈代谢和维系健康的关键物质的排泄物进入毛细血管，在那里，尿素、尿酸、肌氨酸酐等代谢废物形成尿液，身体的必需物如糖、氨基酸、钙、盐被重新吸收回血液中。

Unit 6

Text A

抗生素滥用

有专家担心抗生素的耐药性会使人类处于危险状态，致使人类在感染某些细菌时几乎毫无抵抗之力。世界卫生组织称抗生素耐药性是人类健康的三大威胁之一。

不当使用抗生素导致了对抗生素具有耐药性的细菌群的出现。专家说如果现在不开始着手解决这个问题，本可治愈的感染可能会再度成为危险的病症。美国疾病控制与预防中心的负责人托马斯•弗莱登博士呼吁美国立法者解决这一问题。

"如果我们不改善针对抗生素耐药性这个公共卫生问题的应对机制，我们可能会进入一个后抗生素世界，对某些感染，我们几乎无法进行临床干预。"他说。

专家担心，一种抗生素被使用得越多，它的药效就越低。细菌的遗传突变是一个自然的过程，使细菌对抗生素产生耐药性。但是过量使用药物加速了这个过程。

"最终，泌尿道的细菌将非常具有耐药性。这只是一个例子。还有不同细菌引起的皮肤感染、肺部感染，由于这些细菌的耐药性越来越强，人们遇到的疾病问题也越来越严峻，就像世界上许多地方的肺结核病一样。"一位传染性疾病专家唐纳德•坡茨博士说，"人们为了治疗结核病，这样的抗生素用一点，那样的也用一点，结果结核病菌产生了耐药性。"

"全世界范围内我们都能遇到耐药性问题，可能在世界的不同地方不同药物有不同的耐药性，"他说，"通过快捷的旅游，人们能把这些耐药性细菌传给任何地方的任何人。"

专家说解决办法在于教育病人和医生在没有必要用抗生素时，避免使用抗生素。

Text B

阑尾炎

阑尾是一段位于大肠起始端的、细小的管状结构，也可被称为结肠。它位于右下腹，接近小肠和大肠交界处。

所谓的阑尾炎就是指发生在阑尾的炎症。它常见于二十岁到三十岁的人，但年岁很轻或年老的人也可患此病。男性患者略多于女性。

阑尾炎的发作通常与阑尾管腔阻塞有关。阑尾管腔阻塞以后，常常会引起管腔内压力升高，血液循环受阻和感染。如果阻塞得不到及时的处理，就会导致阑尾管壁坏死甚至破裂。

通常情况下，导致阑尾管腔阻塞的是粪便以及由消化道中的细菌或者病毒而导致的淋巴小结增生。

阑尾炎的症状是多样的，最典型的症状就是转移性右下腹疼痛，多开始于脐周，然后转移至右下腹。该疼痛常常在 6 到 12 小时后会逐渐加剧，甚至会变得很糟糕。疼痛开始后不久可出现恶心和呕吐。通常还会引起发热，但在疾病早期高热者很少。右下腹可出现压痛，扣诊时若手突然放松，可引起反跳痛。

由于阑尾炎的症状类似其他疼痛，这就给医生的诊断增加了难度。在阑尾的解剖位置有某些变化时，疼痛和压痛会引起误诊。若阑尾在盲肠的侧面或后面，压痛可在右侧。若阑尾位于骨盆深部，此时只能通过直肠或骨盆检查方可发现压痛。即使如此，压痛也不易被发现。若由于内脏移位或在胚胎期肠管没有正常旋转，阑尾位于左面时，症状将出现在左方。

外科切除阑尾的手术称为阑尾切除术，它是根治阑尾炎的最有效方法。术前，医生会给病人使用抗生素来预防可能发生的腹膜炎。一般情况下，医生将麻醉病人，然后开腹或者在腹腔镜下切除 4 英寸阑尾。如果病人伴有腹膜炎，医生将会进行腹腔冲洗以去除脓液。

阑尾切除术后，一般需要几个星期病人才能完全康复。在此期间医生一般会嘱咐病人避免重体力劳动，并会给其开一些镇痛药物。如果病人接受的是腹腔镜手术，康复起来可能会快一些，但是在术后 4 到 6 个星期内，仍然应限制重体力劳动。很多得到阑尾炎治疗的病人都康复得很好。

Text C

便秘

便秘是消化系统中常见的健康问题之一，其表现为排便次数减少，粪便干结，或者排便困难，有时甚至好几天都不排便。

即使不是天天排便，也不能就此下结论说就是便秘。判断是便秘的话，还应该有以下表现：

• 粪便干结且一周内排便次数少于 3 次；

• 排便困难经常发作；

• 腹胀或其他腹部不适。

要进一步理解什么是便秘，那就要了解结肠或者说大肠是怎样运转的。当食物残渣随着肠蠕动进入大肠后，其中一部分水分被大肠吸收，形成粪便。粪便随着肠蠕动到达直肠，之后就变成了固体，因为大部分的水被吸收了。

若大肠吸收的水分过多或者肠蠕动减慢使粪便在肠道中停留时间过长，就会导致便秘。结果大便变得干燥坚硬。通常情况下，引起便秘的因素有：

• 水分摄入不足；

• 食物中缺少纤维；

• 没有养成良好的排便习惯；

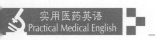
- 年龄；

- 缺乏运动；

- 怀孕；

- 疾病。

当发生便秘的时候，你会感到排便比平时更困难。因为一个或者更多的原因，排便变得更加困难。比如，排便的次数减少，或者无效（感觉排便不尽）。

大多数患有便秘的人不必过分担心，只有少数便秘的人存在严重的医学问题。如果你已经有两个星期以上没有排便了，那就要去医院就诊，以确诊病因并及时治疗。如果便秘是由结肠癌引起的，早诊断、早治疗就显得非常重要。

便秘的诊断通常依赖于你的病史和物理检查。医生首先会想办法确定你的小肠或者直肠有没有阻塞（肠梗阻），然后确定激素水平是否正常，比如是否存在甲状腺功能减退或者电解质失衡。医生还会核实你的药物使用情况，这些药物可能是引发你便秘的原因。

如果便秘不是由于医学问题引起的，就可以通过饮食来调节，比如多喝水，多吃一些纤维素含量高的食物。纤维素可以从大量的蔬菜、水果、面食中获得以及增加饮食中亚麻油的含量。这些常规的非处方通便方法被人们忽视，原因可能是这些通便方法导致肠蠕动变得有依赖性。灌肠可作为一种医学治疗方法来解除便秘。然而，灌肠通常只用于由直肠原因引起的便秘，而非作用于整个肠道系统。

Unit 7

Text A

让我休息

折断的骨头的医学术语为骨折。骨折有很多不同的类型。

骨折只发生在一处地方时被称为单处骨折。你也许听过线形骨折，那是一种微小得像发丝似的单处骨折。当骨头完全被折断分离时被称为完全骨折。当骨头的两处或两处以上被折断时就被称为多处骨折。还有一种类型叫青枝骨折，这种骨折就像一根小树枝被折弯了却没有断一样。这种骨折多发生在孩子身上。另一种类型为开放性骨折或复合骨折，是指骨头暴露在了皮肤之外。这是非常严重的，除了骨头的损坏还伴随着开放性伤口被感染的危险。

身体发生骨折时还会有许多伴随症状。你也许会感到轻微的头疼，或感到胃部不适。受伤严重的病人会出现休克现象，出现冷、晕眩、思维不清等症状。休克需要立刻引起注意。若仅仅感觉骨头疼痛，则通常没有生命危险。

骨折的治疗取决于骨折的类型。医生要通过 X 照片来了解骨折的情况以及骨折的准确位置。严重骨折需要通过手术用金属板或螺丝钉把折断的骨头固定在一起。接着，医生会在病人骨折部位打上模具。在骨头愈合期间也可用弹力绷带将骨折部位固定。一般模具会固定一至两个月。在一些病例中，塑料夹板或金属甲板被用来代替模具控制骨折部位的移动。医生认为出现骨折情况要立刻治疗是因为医生要立刻止血否则会引起病人的神经损坏。而且骨头有自愈的特性，所以也要确保接骨部位正确。

需要补充钙和维生素 D 来帮助骨头生长，以达到足够的强度。通过锻炼增强骨骼强度也能避免骨折的发生。在运动中戴上安全保护用品，如护肘、护腿等是不错的方式。如果你认为这些太拘束，那就尝试戴模具吧！

Text B

急救

急救是在疾病或伤害最初发作时提供的紧急照顾。在专业医务人员到来之前，通常由外行人员给病人或伤员实施急救。某些疾病或小伤可能不需要进一步医疗救助。一般说来，急救包括一系列救生技巧。每个人经过培训后，都可以用极少量设备来操作这些技巧。

根据英国国家统计办公室调查，家庭意外事故和伤害事件前五位为摔倒、碰撞、割伤和撕伤、异物，以及搬动家具等情况下发生的过度用力。

美国急诊医师学会提出了以下预防医疗紧急情况的办法。

• 每年定期体检，常规锻炼。

• 确定自己是否存在有生命受到威胁的风险，确保健康。遵循医生减少风险因素的建议，如不要吸烟；如有吸烟习惯，则戒掉。

• 把所有药物放在孩子拿不到的地方。

• 把所有有毒物质存放在孩子拿不到的地方。

• 谨慎驾驶，注意天气和路况。车上所有乘客应系好安全带。

• 在喝酒和服用药物后不要操纵交通工具。

• 认真阅读药品的警示标签，弄清服用该药物是否损坏驾驶和操作机械的能力。

人们认为某些技能在提供急救时是基本的。尤其是在治疗某些不太严重的伤害时必须实施急救的 "ABC"。ABC 代表气道 (Airway)、呼吸 (Breathing) 和循环 (Circulation)。 首先要注意确保气道通畅。窒息是威胁生命的紧急情况。在评价气道情况之后，最初的急救人员应确定通气程度，如有必要应提供氧气。一般通过检查颈动脉来评估血液循环状况，由此确定是否进行心肺复苏。

一些机构用 "3B"，即呼吸 (Breathing)、流血 (Bleeding) 和骨骼 (Bones) 来表示相同的急救措施优先秩序。ABC 和 3B 都是分步实施，而某些情况要求同时考虑两个步骤。 如对停止呼吸没有脉搏的人应同时进行人工呼吸和胸部压迫。

一些急救措施是需要经过训练的，对常见损伤和创伤的处理办法也可以经过训练学会。例如，对割伤和擦伤，可以用冷水冲洗。可以用纱布稳固但轻柔地压着伤口止血。如果血液渗出，就用更多纱布，保持压力。

应记住紧急情况下可拨打 120。这是中国的急救电话。在家里和汽车上配备急救包也

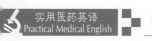

非常重要。急救包里应该有急救指南。阅读急救指南，学会使用急救包里的物品很重要。这样如有紧急情况出现，你便有所准备。

Text C

骨折

若有外力施加在骨骼上，骨骼便有可能出问题。如果骨骼不能承受这些外力，就会发生骨折。骨折发生时，骨骼将失去完整性，骨骼结构被破坏。

根据发生部位和外观等特点，骨折有许多种类。如果折骨周围的皮肤没有破损，被称为闭合骨折。开放骨折时，皮肤破损，暴露骨头，伤口更易受感染。如果骨骼完全折断，被称为完全骨折；如果是部分折断则被称为非完全骨折或青枝骨折。若骨骼承受长期重复活动带来的压力而破裂，被称为压力性骨折。根据骨折线形状不同，分为横形骨折、斜形骨折和螺旋形骨折。如果骨头折成许多片，被称为粉碎性骨折。事实上，骨折可能为单一种类，也可能同时包括多种骨折。

一般说来，骨折会导致疼痛，肿大，有时因内出血出现瘀伤。受伤区域不能承受重力或压力，移动时会产生剧烈疼痛。折骨周围的软组织也可能受伤。若患处脉搏丧失，骨折周围或其以下部位可能会出现麻木或瘫痪。

可通过对患处进行体格检查和放射检查来诊断骨折。然而，某些类型的骨折很难通过放射检查被发现。在这种情况下，医生会对病人做诊断性的影像分析，如计算机断层扫描、磁共振成像或骨骼扫描。开放骨折需要进行另外的医学化验检查以确定是否有失血或存在感染风险。

对手、臂、足、腿部位的骨折进行的首要治疗包括给肢体原位上夹板、抬高受伤肢体、冰敷受伤区域等。固定患处对控制最初疼痛极有帮助。对于颈部和背部损伤，最初参与治疗的急救人员或护理人员可以将伤员置于长形木板上，戴上项领，以保护脊髓免受潜在的损伤。

骨折手术在很大程度上取决于折骨类型和骨折部位。外科医生对折骨进行处理，使骨头位置复原，再安上石膏等固定位置。有时，折骨需要插入金属来固定位置。根据骨折情况的不同，有时这些金属是永久安放不再取出；有时只是暂时安放，在折骨完全愈合后一段时间再通过手术取出。

Unit 8

Text A

佛罗伦斯·南丁格尔

每年的 5 月 12 日是国际护士节，它是为了纪念护士职业的创始人、英国护理学先驱和现代护理教育奠基人佛罗伦斯·南丁格尔而设立的。

佛罗伦斯·南丁格尔于 1820 年 5 月 12 日出生于意大利佛罗伦萨一个富裕和受过良好教育的家庭。在孩提时代，她就有一颗仁慈和充满同情的心，会细心地护理那些受了伤的小动物。1850 年，她不顾家人的反对，前往德国学习护理。

1854 年至 1856 年，英、法、土耳其联军与沙皇俄国在克里米亚交战，南丁格尔奔赴战地并建立了第一所我们现在所说的战地医院：卫生、安全、设备齐全。她对伤员不知疲倦的照顾誉满全球。在战地医院，她每夜都手提油灯巡视伤病员，被称为"提灯女神"。1857 年，她促成了皇家陆军卫生委员会的建立，同年还开办了陆军军医学校。1860 年，南丁格尔利用公众捐款，在英国圣托马斯医院内创建了第一所正规护士学校——佛罗伦斯·南丁格尔护士学校。她撰写的《医院笔记》《护理笔记》等著作成为医院管理、护士教育的基础教材。1901 年，南丁格尔因操劳过度，双目失明。1907 年，为表彰南丁格尔对医疗工作的卓越贡献，英国国王授予她功绩勋章，她成为英国首位获此殊荣的妇女。晚年的南丁格尔致力于提高公众健康水平，提高医院护理标准，把护理事业带出困境并使之成为专业性强且受人尊敬的职业。1910 年，南丁格尔逝世，享年 90 岁。遵照她的遗嘱，未举行国葬。

为纪念南丁格尔对护理事业所做的贡献，国际护士理事会在 1912 年将她的生日定为国际护士节，以激励护士继承和发扬护理事业的光荣传统，用"爱心、耐心、细心、责任心"对待每一位病人，做好护理工作。她的生日也成为英美国家各医院"全国医院周"的核心内容，每个医院都会举办特别的展览、讨论会和宣传活动。

Text B

白血病

白血病是一种造血系统的恶性疾病，俗称"血癌"。其特点是骨髓及其他造血组织中有大量白血病细胞无限制地增生，并进入外周血液及器官组织，而正常血细胞的制造则被明显抑制。

白血病有多种类型，主要以血液内异常的血细胞类型来划分。临床学和病理学上把白血病分为急性白血病和慢性白血病。此外，白血病也可根据白细胞受影响的类型分为淋巴细胞白血病和骨髓细胞白血病。

目前尚未完全确定白血病的病因。研究发现，白血病可能与辐射、部分化学物质（包括化学药物）、病毒感染和遗传因素等有关。放射核素对动物和人类的致白血病作用已经得到肯定。一次大剂量或多次小剂量的放射核素照射均可引起白血病。国际卫生组织已经把苯定为强致癌物质。长期吸入苯会破坏人体的循环系统和造血机能，导致白血病。近些年来，日常生活中的苯主要来自建筑装饰中大量使用的化工原料，如涂料、木器漆、胶黏剂及各种有机溶剂。

通过产生大量不成熟的白细胞来取代正常的骨髓细胞从而损害骨髓，会导致以下症状：

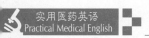
- 凝血过程中缺少血小板，白血病病人可能更容易被擦伤、流血过多。
- 白细胞（通常也被称为免疫细胞）可能被抑制或功能紊乱。这将影响病人的免疫能力。
- 红细胞不足会导致贫血，引起病人呼吸困难。

通常临床上可观察到以下相关症状：

- 发热、畏寒、盗汗和其他一些类似流感的症状；
- 体弱疲劳；
- 牙龈肿痛或出血；
- 神经学症状，如头痛；
- 肝脾肿大；
- 频繁感染；
- 骨骼或关节疼痛（例如膝盖、臀部或肩部疼痛）；
- 头晕；
- 恶心；
- 淋巴结肿胀，特别是颈部和腋窝的淋巴肿胀；
- 腹泻；
- 面色苍白；
- 不适；
- 体重减轻。

以上所有症状都有可能源于其他疾病，为了确诊是否为白血病，需要进行血液检查、骨髓穿刺检查等。

白血病的治疗取决于白血病的类型、不同白血病细胞的特征、病人疾病的严重程度、病人的治疗史以及病人的年龄和身体状况等。病人可以接受化疗、生物疗法、放射疗法或者骨髓移植等。如果病人的脾脏肿大，医生可能会建议采用外科手术将它摘除。有些病人需要接受综合治疗。

Text C

艾滋病

人们受到艾滋病毒的威胁已经超过二十年，已经有成千上万人死于艾滋病。艾滋病已成为当今世界所面临的最大问题之一。大家都应该了解有关艾滋病的基本知识。

艾滋病 (AIDS) 是获得性免疫缺陷综合征的简称，是由人类免疫缺陷病毒 (HIV) 所引起的致命性慢性传染病。该病主要通过性接触和血液传播，病毒主要侵犯和破坏辅助性 T 淋巴细胞，使机体细胞免疫功能受损，最后并发各种严重的机会性感染和肿瘤。

艾滋病的症状因内脏机能和肿瘤部位的不同而不同。常见的艾滋病症状有以下几个方面。

- 一般症状：持续发热、虚弱、盗汗、全身浅表淋巴结肿大、体重下降等；

- 呼吸道症状：长期咳嗽、胸痛、呼吸困难、严重时痰中带血等；
- 消化道症状：厌食、恶心、呕吐、腹泻、严重时便血等；
- 神经系统症状：头晕、头痛、反应迟钝、智力减退、精神失常、抽搐、偏瘫、痴呆等；
- 皮肤和黏膜损害：弥漫性丘疹、带状疱疹、口腔和咽部黏膜炎症及溃烂等；
- 多种恶性肿瘤：如位于体表的卡波西氏肉瘤，可见红色或紫红色的斑疹、丘疹和浸润性肿块。

由此可见，艾滋病的症状是非常复杂的。

诊断是否有艾滋病毒感染可以通过检定抗疾病蛋白或血液里抗体的表现来进行。有两种不同类型的抗体试验可供选择：酶联免疫分析（ELISA）和免疫着色。

避免某些高风险行为可减少感染艾滋病毒的概率：

- 避免性滥交；
- 每次性行为都使用安全套；
- 使用静脉注射时，不要与其他人共用针头；
- 医疗保健工作者应严格遵循预防措施（建立感染控制程序，避免接触患者的体液）；
- 计划怀孕的女性，最好预先做一个关于艾滋病毒的测试，特别是有过高风险艾滋病毒感染行为的人群。艾滋病毒感染呈阳性的孕妇需要接受特别的产前护理和药物治疗，以降低艾滋病毒传给新生婴儿的风险。

自 20 世纪 90 年代中期以来，艾滋病的防治工作已经得到很大改善，但到目前为止仍然没有根治此病的方法。总的治疗原则为抗感染、抗肿瘤、杀灭或抑制艾滋病毒、增强机体免疫机能。

Unit 9

Text A

儿童肥胖

过去二十年以来，儿童肥胖者的数量几乎增加了三倍，因此，这成了一个值得讨论的重要话题。遗憾的是，对很多人来说，儿童肥胖是一个敏感的问题而且这个问题经常被忽略。

肥胖对健康的不利影响有很多，会增加患心脏病、高血压、2 型糖尿病和各种癌症的概率。已从 6 岁小孩的病例中发现代谢的问题。

在大多数情况下，一名超重儿童可以通过改变饮食习惯和生活方式来达到减肥的目的。大多数孩子把大量的时间花在了玩电脑游戏、看电视、上网冲浪上并用了很长的时间做作业。

治疗儿童肥胖非常困难，而有效减肥并保持减肥效果的人数非常少。

预防是策略，教育是关键。需要教育小孩什么是肥胖、肥胖产生的原因、肥胖的危险性以及健康的饮食方式。此外，教育小孩如何烹饪也很重要，要避免依赖外卖和快餐。当然，还要特别强调锻炼的重要性。

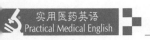

中国政府当然清楚需要采取措施。中国疾病预防控制中心曾向中国儿童及其父母发布了健康饮食指南，试图降低日益增长的儿童肥胖率。

教育部前部长周济曾明确要求，学校应该保证每天至少一小时的体育锻炼时间。

但最终，家庭应负起责任。在家提倡合理均衡的饮食，多做运动，少看电视和少玩电脑游戏，这些都会为孩子树立良好的榜样。

在英国国家肥胖论坛上，儿童肥胖是否该被当作一个儿童保护问题曾引发了人们激烈的争论。这是考虑到由忽视引起肥胖而导致的后果与由忽视引起营养不良而导致的后果一样严重。这肯定是引人沉思的事情。

Text B

肥胖

肥胖是指机体脂肪过多，通常被认为是一种不健康的生理状态。医学上，肥胖有别于体重超重，因为肌肉、骨骼、脂肪和体液均能使体重增加。肥胖是因为长期过多摄入脂肪或热量而导致的。

测量体重是否超重的方法有很多。但健康保健人员认为，采用体重指数是最恰当的方法。体重指数的计算公式是：BMI = 体重 / 身高的二次方，其中体重的单位是千克；身高的单位是米。世界卫生组织在 1997 年给出了一个参数值；若 BMI 小于 18.5，则表示体重过轻；若 BMI 介于 18.5 ～ 24.9，则表示体重正常；若 BMI 介于 25.0 ～ 29.9，则表示体重超重；若 BMI 介于 30.0 ～ 39.9，则表示肥胖；若 BMI 是 40.0 或大于 40.0，则表示严重肥胖。要想不肥胖，能量平衡是很重要的。

肥胖与许多因素有关，如能量、活动、环境、基因、家族史、健康状况、药物、情绪、年龄、吸烟、怀孕以及睡眠。当从食物中摄入的能量与工作、呼吸、消化等生理活动消耗的能量相同时，就达到了能量平衡状态；若摄入的能量比消耗的能量多，体重就会增加；反之，体重就会减少。因此，身体长期摄入过多能量就会引起肥胖。

许多因素会引起肥胖。现代社会中，越来越多的人根本不进行身体锻炼。除了每天 8 小时的工作以及加班以外，大多数人的业余时间都是在看电视或坐在电脑前浏览网页或与陌生人闲聊。实际上，每天在电视前坐两小时就可致肥胖。其他因素也减少了运动时间。人们宁愿开车上班也不走路去办公室。现代科技为人们带来便利的同时也减少了人们的活动需求，因此人体脂肪的燃烧也减少了。

环境改变着人们的生活习惯。拥挤的居住环境减少了社区公园和散步的场所。大量可供选择的、高脂肪高热量的食物也导致越来越多的人肥胖。

激素和药物也会改变人们的饮食和生活习惯。药物可能减缓能量消耗，增加食欲或使水潴留在人体内。人们承受情感压力时，可能吃得更多。随着年龄的增长，机体会失去很多肌肉，因此能量消耗会减慢，从而使更多的能量堆积在体内。

肥胖会增加人们患上以下疾病的风险：

- 高血压；

- 骨质疏松症；

- 2 型糖尿病；

- 冠心病；

- 中风；

- 胆囊炎；

- 失眠和呼吸系统疾病；

- 癌症，如子宫内膜癌、乳腺癌、结肠癌。

然而，肥胖者若体重减轻 5% 至 10% 就可远离这些疾病。

Text C

压力

一位衣着讲究的白领对她的朋友说："这些日子我觉得很压抑。"这让她的朋友很吃惊。"因为工作让我很有压力。"

许多人调研过压力。那么究竟什么是压力？汉斯·赛利（Hans Selye）在 1936 年第一次使用了这个词语。汉斯把"压力"定义为"机体对变化的不明确的反应"。也有人把"压力"定义为"机体应对变化时产生的一种情感"。字典上把"压力"定义为"一种生理、心理和情绪的张力"或"个体意识到需求超出个人和社会的能力范围时产生的情况或情感"。医学上认为压力会在生理上和心理上破坏体内平衡。

应对压力时，人们的情绪、心理和生理都会产生变化。医学通过对神经系统和激素的刺激研究可以解释压力产生的基本原因。下丘脑发出信号使得肾上腺产生更多的肾上腺激素和皮质激素进入血液，而这些激素会加快心跳和呼吸，增高血压，加快新陈代谢。血管进一步扩张，瞳孔增大，肝脏释放更多储存的血糖进入血液，汗液分泌增多。短时间的轻微压力有助于人处理紧急事件，可以使人表现得更好。然而，面对过多的压力，如果处理不好，或者不能从压力中很快恢复，就会引起很多问题。

人们无法避免现代社会快速的工作和生活所产生的压力，但是可以学会接受压力，在压力下生活。首先，要学会辨认压力产生的症状。压力最先影响的是内心情绪。压力使人们觉得焦急、恐慌、压抑甚至特别忧虑。然后人们对周围事物变得很敏感，容易从工作中分心，以自我为中心。如果压力没能得到控制，日益累积，人们就会觉得乏力、胃部不适、胸闷、失眠，甚至恶心呕吐。其次，应该了解怎样控制压力。压力伴随着变化和挑战的发生。重新看看日程安排，放弃不太重要的事情，做出最优的选择。对工作成就要有比较现实的预期。要有充足的高质量的睡眠。最后，要尽量多了解产生压力的原因。好和不好的事件都可能引起压力。一旦出现有压力的征兆，尽量找出是由什么引起的：工作、学习、

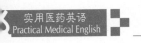

家庭、社会、生活习惯还是环境。

人们都知道在巨大压力下生活的人容易有不利于健康的行为和形成不利于健康的习惯。因此，压力会损害健康。压力有多种表现形式，也会影响各个年龄段的人。时间和空间是治疗压力最好的良药。

Unit 10

Text A

关注心理健康

每年的 10 月 10 日是世界心理卫生日。本年度的主题是关注类似糖尿病和癌症的慢性物理疾病与心理健康之间的关系。

世界卫生组织称，超过 4.5 亿的人患有轻微心理健康疾病，最常见的是抑郁症和精神分裂症。心理健康专家还将其他一些问题列入这个范畴，例如影响数百万人的药物和酒精的滥用。

艾伦娜·伯杰是世界心理卫生联盟的成员。1992 年，这家总部位于美国的组织举办了第一届世界心理卫生日的活动。

伯杰称，心理健康问题在贫穷国家是极为严重的，这些地区缺乏解决心理健康问题的资源。

她说："这是个巨大的问题，世界卫生组织将心理健康列为一个被忽视的问题。在发展中国家，高达 85% 的人没有接受心理健康治疗的途径，这类地区不存在该类治疗服务，有着巨大的人员需求，而且，许多患心理疾病的群体都遭受了严重的歧视。"

专家称，大约有一半的心理健康问题在人们 15 岁之前就会首次暴露。发展中国家是年轻人所占比例最高的，这也意味着，这些国家也是心理健康治疗资源最匮乏的国家。

世界卫生组织称，许多中低收入国家每 100 万到 400 万的人口中只有一个儿童心理医生。

在全球范围内，抑郁是心理健康的头号问题，也是导致功能障碍的主要因素。世界卫生组织估计，2002 年超过 1 亿 5400 万的人患有抑郁症。

但是，伯杰认为其他方面的疾病经常得到更多的重视。

她说："人们对于传染性疾病关注得更多，而没有注意源自心理健康问题的各类功能障碍。人们无法全身心投入工作以赚取收入就是一种功能障碍。它还会对家庭成员产生很大的影响。"

伯杰称，她所在的组织和世界卫生组织正在督促各国政府把心理健康医疗列入他们的发展目标中，这将会极大地改善全球心理健康治疗和服务。

她说："在目前情况下，患有精神和心理障碍的人们应该被视为一个需要特别支持的弱势群体，他们需要社会的接纳，而不是被排除和忽略。"

Text B

冠心病

心脏把血液泵到全身，每分钟大约跳动 70 次。血液离开心脏后，到达肺部吸收氧气。含氧血液回到心脏，通过动脉网络被输送到全身各个器官。血液通过静脉返回心脏，然后又再次被泵到肺部。这个过程被称为血液循环。

心脏从其表面的血管网络得到血液供应，这些血管网络就是冠状动脉。冠心病是指冠状动脉中脂肪物质堆积，心脏血液供应被阻塞或中断的情况。

如果冠状动脉被部分阻塞，会产生胸痛（心绞痛）。如果冠状动脉被完全阻塞，会导致心脏病发作（心肌梗塞）。心脏病发作会对心肌产生永久性损害；如果不及时治疗，会导致生命危险。如果病人察觉心脏病发作，应该拨打 120 以获得迅速的医疗救助。

冠心病病人可能会出现心悸。心悸在心脏跳动不规则时，或心脏跳动力度比正常状态更大时产生。应该意识到，心悸并非一定和冠心病有联系，所以，如果有心悸不要过度焦虑。然而不管怎样，到医生处做一下检查最好。

有冠心病的人还会发生心力衰竭。心脏太虚弱，不能把血液泵到全身，导致体液在肺部聚集，使肺部呼吸困难。心力衰竭可能突然发生（急性心力衰竭），也可能经过长时间后发生（慢性心力衰竭）。

以下人群患冠心病的概率会明显提高：

- 吸烟者；
- 高血压病人；
- 胆固醇水平较高者；
- 缺乏定期体力锻炼的人；
- 血栓症病人；
- 糖尿病病人。

冠心病不能被治愈，但近来新药的研究和开发出现了进展，手术治疗效果有明显提高，意味着冠心病能得到更加有效的控制。在恰当地进行治疗后，冠心病症状能减少，心脏功能能得到改善。

如果由于动脉粥样化导致血管变得十分狭窄，或者药物不能控制症状，这时可能需要进行外科手术来打开或替换被阻塞的动脉。冠状动脉搭桥术、心脏移植和激光手术等外科手术可以用来治疗被阻塞的动脉。

预防冠心病的最好办法是确保低密度脂蛋白 (LDL) 水平较低和高密度脂蛋白 (HDL) 水平较高。可通过许多方式预防冠心病，如：

- 健康均衡的饮食；
- 更多体力锻炼；

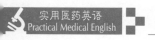

- 戒烟；
- 减少酒精摄入量；
- 控制血压；
- 控制糖尿病；
- 服用医生开出的药物。

Text C

高血压

全世界约有 10 亿人患有高血压，它是导致发病和死亡的一个主要原因。许多人并没有意识到他们患有高血压。因此，这种疾病有时被称为"无声杀手"。在人们能观察到高血压的损害后果（如中风、心肌梗塞、肾脏功能紊乱、视力问题等）之前，高血压往往是没有症状的。

高血压被定义为血压的异常升高。收缩压和舒张压数值都应被注意。根据最近的美国全国诊断指南，可用下表的数值来描述高血压的不同阶段。

高血压最新指南

分　类	收缩压 (mmHg)	舒张压 (mmHg)
正常血压	<120	<80
血压升高	120～129	<80
高血压 1 期	130～139	80～89
高血压 2 期	≥140	≥90

90%～95% 的高血压病人的病因尚不清楚，这种情况被称为原发性高血压。其余 5%～10% 的病人的高血压是由于肾病、内分泌疾病、或其他可确认病因而引发的，这种高血压被称为继发性高血压。

高血压危象指可能导致中风的血压急剧升高。血压过度增高将损害血管。心脏不能维持足够的血液循环。高血压危象有高血压急症和高血压亚急症两类。高血压急症的体征和症状包括血压升高、严重头痛、严重焦虑和呼吸短促。高血压亚急症病人会出现肺水肿、脑肿或脑出血、心脏病发作、中风等威胁生命的体征和症状。

医生不能确定大多数高血压病例的病因，但是人们现已公认有几种情况会使血压升高，如肥胖、酗酒、高血压家族史、盐摄入过多、衰老等。体力锻炼过少、钾和钙摄取不足也可能会使血压升高。

高血压一般不会有症状。大多数人因其他原因就医时才被告知他们患有高血压。如果不经治疗，高血压会损害心脏、大脑、肾或眼睛。会导致冠心病、中风和肾脏衰竭等问题。非常高的血压会导致头痛、视力问题、恶心和呕吐。

高血压的治疗取决于病人血压的高度，病人是否有糖尿病等其他健康问题，病人是否已有器官损伤。医生也会考虑病人患上其他疾病，特别是心脏病的可能性。大多数高血压病人用抗高血压药物进行治疗，或常用降低心脏输出量的药物进行治疗。血管扩张药物会降低全身血管阻力，也被用来治疗高血压。

  人们可以采用健康的生活方式来降低血压。如果这些方式不起作用，则可能需要服用药物。有助于预防高血压的生活方式包括：

- 减肥；
- 减少盐的摄入量；
- 锻炼；
- 限制酒精的摄入量；
- 每天从饮食中摄入 3 500 mg 的钾。新鲜的未被加工的完整食物中钾的含量最高，如肉、鱼、无脂或低脂奶制品以及多数水果和蔬菜。

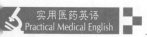

6. Word Learning Booster

Unit One

Part 2   Listening and Speaking

Talking About Your College Life

pharmaceutical /ˌfɑ:mə'sju:tɪkəl/ *adj.* 制药的

physiology /ˌfɪzi'ɒlədʒɪ/ *n.* 生理学

sophomore /'sɒfəmɔ:/ *n.* 大学二年级学生

fundamental /ˌfʌndə'mentl/ *n.* 基本原则

surgical /'sɜ:dʒɪkəl/ *adj.* 外科的

sterilization /sterɪlaɪ'zeɪʃ ən/ *n.* 杀菌

institution /ˌɪnstɪ'tju:ʃ ən/ *n.* 公共机构

Part 3   Reading Comprehension

Chemistry Is Life

tissue /'tɪʃu:/ *n.* 组织

soluble /'sɒljʊbl/ *adj.* 可溶的

gland /ɡlænd/ *n.* 腺体

dioxide /daɪ'ɒksaɪd/ *n.* 二氧化物

prescribe /prɪs'kraɪb/ *vt.* 给……开药

antiseptic /æntɪ'septɪk/ *n.* 消毒剂

hinder /'hɪndə/ *v.* 防止

nylon /'naɪlɒn/ *n.* 尼龙

metallic /mɪ'tælɪk/ *adj.* 金属的

alloy /'ælɒɪ/ *n.* 合金

Body Structure and Function

anatomy /ə'nætəmi/ *n.* 解剖学

homeostasis /ˌhəumɪə'steɪsɪs/ *n.* 动态平衡

complicated /'kɒmplɪkeɪtɪd/ *adj.* 复杂的

microscopic /maɪkrə'skɒpɪk/ *adj.* 精微的

identity /aɪ'dentɪti/ *n.* 特性

fertilize /'fɜ:tɪlaɪz/ *vt.* 使受精

definition /ˌdefɪ'nɪʃ ən/ *n.* 定义

intercellular /ˌɪntə'seljʊlə/ *adj.* 细胞间的

epithelial /ˌepɪ'θi:lɪəl/ *adj.* 上皮的

lining /'laɪnɪŋ/ *n.* 内层

skeletal /'skelɪtl/ *adj.* 骨骼的

muscular /'mʌskjʊlə/ *adj.* 肌肉的

endocrine /'endəukrɪn/ *n.* 内分泌

cardiovascular /ˌkɑ:diəu'væskjʊlə/ *adj.* 心脏血管的

lymphatic /lɪm'fætɪk/ *adj.* 淋巴的

respiratory /rɪ'spɪrətəri/ *adj.* 呼吸的

digestive /daɪ'dʒestɪv/ *adj.* 消化的

urinary /'jʊərɪnəri/ *adj.* 泌尿的

reproductive /ˌri:prə'dʌktɪv/ *adj.* 生殖的

physiological /ˌfɪzɪə'lɒdʒɪkəl/ *adj.* 生理学的

psychological /ˌsaɪkə'lɒdʒɪkəl/ *adj.* 心理学的

survival /sə'vaɪvəl/ *n.* 生存

constancy /'kɒnstənsi/ *n.* 恒久不变的状态

Life Process

metabolize /mə'tæbəlaɪz/ *v.* 使新陈代谢

infancy /'ɪnfənsi/ *n.* 幼年

maturity /mə'tʃʊərɪti/ *n.* 成熟

adulthood /'ædʌlthʊd/ *n.* 成人期

metabolism /mə'tæbəlɪzəm/ *n.* 新陈代谢

differentiation /ˌdɪfə,renʃɪ'eɪʃ ən/ *n.* 分化

respiration /ˌrespə'reɪʃ ən/ *n.* 呼吸

digestion /daɪ'dʒestʃ ən/ *n.* 消化

interrelated /ɪntərɪ'leɪtɪd/ *adj.* 相关的

disruption /dɪs'rʌpʃ ən/ *n.* 破坏

component /kəm'pəunənt/ *n.* 成分

integrity /ɪn'teɡrɪti/ *n.* 完整

catabolism /kə'tæbəlɪzəm/ *n.* 分解代谢

irritability /ɪrɪtə'bɪlətɪ/ *n.* 过敏

stimulus /'stɪmjuləs/ *n.* 刺激

cellular /'seljʊlə/ *adj.* 细胞的

molecule /'mɒlɪkju:l/ *n.* 分子

diaphragm /'daɪəfræm/ *n.* 横膈膜

replacement /rɪ'pleɪsmənt/ *n.* 代替

anabolic /ə'næbəlɪk/ *adj.* 合成代谢的

distinctive /dɪs'tɪŋktɪv/ *adj.* 有特色的

excretion /ɪk'skri:ʃ ən/ *n.* 排泄

toxic /'tɒksɪk/ *adj.* 有毒的

incompatible /ˌɪnkəm'pætəbl/ *adj.* 不调和的

nutrient /'nju:triənt/ *n.* 营养物

Unit Two

Part 2   Listening and Speaking

Introducing the Hospital

physician /fɪ'zɪʃən/ *n.* 医师，内科医师

surgeon /'sɜ:dʒən/ *n.* 外科医生

dentist /'dentɪst/ *n.* 牙科医生

Consulting a Doctor

midwife /'mɪdwaɪf/ *n.* 助产士

pharmacy /'fɑ:məsi/ *n.* 药房

injection /ɪn'dʒekʃən/ *n.* 注射

transfusion /træns'fju:ʒən/ *n.* 输液

Part 3   Reading Comprehension

You Are What You Eat

carbohydrate /,kɑ:bəʊ'haɪdreɪt/ *n.* 碳水化合物

protein /'prəʊti:n/ *n.* 蛋白质

fluid /'flu:ɪd/ *n.* 流体

organic /ɔ:'gænik/ *adj.* 有机的

carbon /'kɑ:bən/ *n.* 碳

hydrogen /'haɪdrədʒən/ *n.* 氢

oxygen /'ɒksɪdʒən/ *n.* 氧

atom /'ætəm/ *n.* 原子

starch /stɑ:tʃ/ *n.* 淀粉

ester /'estə/ *n.* 酯

nitrogen /'naɪtrədʒən/ *n.* 氮

protoplasm /'prəʊtəplæzəm/ *n.* 原生质

tract /trækt/ *n.*(连通身体组织或器官的) 道

infection /in'fekʃən/ *n.* 感染

contagious /kən'teɪdʒəs/ *adj.* 传染性的

virus /'vaɪərəs/ *n.* 病毒

recur /rɪ'kɜ:/ *vi.* 复发

drainage /'dreinidʒ/ *n.* 引流

typically /'tɪpɪkli/ *adv.* 通常

sinus /'saɪnəs/ *n.* 窦

bronchitis /brɒŋ'kaɪtɪs/ *n.* 支气管炎

asthma /'æsmə/ *n.* 哮喘

chronic /'krɒnɪk/ *adj.* 慢性的

emphysema /,emfɪ'si:mə/ *n.* 肺气肿

mechanism /'mekənɪzəm/ *n.* 机制

Common Cold

antibiotic /,æntɪbaɪ'ɒtɪk/ *n.* 抗生素

allergic /ə'lɜ:dʒɪk/ *adj.* 过敏的

bacterial /bæk'tɪərɪəl/ *adj.* 细菌的

complication /,kɒmplɪ'keɪʃən/ *n.* 并发症

decongestant /,di:kən'dʒestənt/ *n.* 减充血剂

spray /spreɪ/ *n.* 喷雾

pneumonia /nju:'məʊnɪə/ *n.* 肺炎

fungi /'fʌndʒaɪ/ *n.*(fungus 的复数) 真菌

parasite /'pærəsaɪt/ *n.* 寄生虫

subsequently /'sʌbsɪkwəntli/ *adv.* 后来

accompany /ə'kʌmpəni/ *vt.* 伴随

clammy /'klæmi/ *adj.* 湿黏的

fatigue /fə'ti:g/ *n.* 疲劳

culture /'kʌltʃə/ *n.*（细菌）培养

Pneumonia

hospitalization /,hɒspɪtəlaɪ'zeɪʃən/ *n.* 住院治疗

microorganism /,maɪkrəʊ'ɒ:gənɪzəm/ *n.* 微生物

sensitivity /,sensɪ'tɪvɪti/ *n.* 灵敏性

artificial /,ɑ:tɪ'fɪʃəl/ *adj.* 人工的

ventilation /,ventɪ'leɪʃən/ *n.* 流通空气

pleural /'plʊərə/ *adj.* 胸膜的

effusion/ɪ'fju:ʒən/ *n.* 流出物

abscess /'æbses/ *n.* 脓肿

administer /əd'mɪnɪstə/ *vt.* 给予

edema /ɪ'di:mə/ *n.* 浮肿，水肿

imperative /ɪm'perətɪv/ *adj.* 必要的

Unit Three

Part 2   Listening and Speaking

Introducing the Ward

hospitalize /'hɒspɪtlaɪz/ *vt.* 住院

necessity /nɪ'sesɪti/ *n.* 必需品

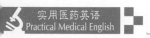
Admitting a Patient

valuables /'væljuəblz/ *n.* 贵重物品

Part 3　Reading Comprehension

CPR

compression /kəm'preʃən/ *n.* 挤压

vital /'vaɪtl/ *adj.* 至关重要的

paramedic /'pærə'medɪk/ *n.* 医护人员

Severe Acute Respiratory Syndrome

coronavirus /kɒrənə'vaɪrəs/ *n.* 冠状病毒

pandemic /pæn'demɪk/ *n.* 流行病

mortality /mɔː'tælətɪ/ *n.* 死亡率

certify /'sɜːtɪfaɪ/ *vt.* 发证书给（某人）

initial /ɪ'nɪʃəl/ *adj.* 最初的

myalgia /maɪ'ældʒə/ *n.* 肌痛

lethargy /'leθədʒi/ *n.* 无生气

gastrointestinal /ˌgæstrəʊɪn'testənl/ *adj.* 胃与肠的

syndrome /'sɪndrəʊm/ *n.* 症状

Bird Flu

avian /'eɪvɪən/ *adj.* 鸟类的 *n.* 鸟

influenza /ˌɪnflu'enzə/ *n.* 流行性感冒

host /həʊst/ *n.* 宿主

platelet /'pleɪtlɪt/ *n.* 血小板

antipyretic /ˌæntɪpaɪ'retɪk/ *n.* 退热剂

supplemental /ˌsʌpli'mentl/ *adj.* 补足的

ventilatory /'ventɪlətərɪ/ *adj.* 通气的

anecdotal /ˌænik'dəʊtl/ *adj.* 传闻的

ribavirin /raɪbə'vaɪərɪn/ *n.* 病毒唑（抗病毒药）

clinician /klɪ'nɪʃən/ *n.* 临床医生

detrimental /ˌdetrɪ'mentl/ *adj.* 有害的

hepatitis /ˌhepə'taɪtɪs/ *n.* 肝炎

immune /ɪ'mjuːn/ *adj.* 免疫的

modulate /'mɒdjʊleɪt/ *vt.* 调节

poultry /'pəʊltri/ *n.* 家禽

mutate /mjuː'teɪt/ *vi.* 变异

vaccine /'væksiːn/ *n.* 疫苗

intestine /ɪn'testɪn/ *n.* 肠

domesticate /də'mestɪkeɪt/ *vt.* 驯养（动物）

saliva /sə'laɪvə/ *n.* 唾液

secretion /si'kriːʃən/ *n.* 分泌物

feces /'fiːsiːz/ *n.* 粪便，排泄物

susceptible /sə'septəbl/ *adj.* 易受影响的

contaminate /kən'tæmɪneɪt/ *vt.* 污染

feed /fiːd/ *n.* 饲料

distress /dɪs'tres/ *n.* 窘迫

prescription /prɪ'skrɪpʃən/ *n.* 处方

resistant /rɪ'zɪstənt/ *adj.* 有耐药性的

Unit Four

Part 3　Reading Comprehension

Traditional Chinese Medicine

herbal /'hɜːbl/ *adj.* 草药的

clinical /'klɪnɪkəl/ *adj.* 临床的

diagnostic /ˌdaɪəg'nɒstɪk/ *adj.* 诊断的

vitality /vaɪ'tælɪti/ *n.* 生命力，活力

diagnosis /ˌdaɪəg'nəʊsɪs/ *n.* 诊断

remedy /'remɪdi/ *n.* 疗法

pharmacological /ˌfɑːməkə'lɒdʒɪkəl/ *adj.* 药理学的

Cerebral Hemorrhage

ingredient /ɪn'griːdiənt/ *n.* 成分

therapeutic /ˌθerə'pjuːtɪk/ *adj.* 治疗的

hemorrhage /'hemərɪdʒ/ *n.* 出血

rupture /'rʌptʃə/ *n.* 破裂

accumulate /ə'kjuːmjʊleɪt/ *vi.* 积聚

membrane /'membreɪn/ *n.* 薄膜

hemisphere /'hemɪsfɪə/ *n.* 半球

intracerebral /ˌɪntrə'serəbrəl/ *adj.* 大脑内的

traumatic /trɔː'mætɪk/ *adj.* 创伤的

tumour /'tjuːmə/ *n.* 瘤

abnormality /ˌæbnɔː'mælɪti/ *n.* 异常性

swelling /'swelɪŋ/ *n.* 肿胀

hematoma /ˌhiːmə'təʊmə/ *n.* 血肿

nausea /'nɔːsiə/ *n.* 恶心

consciousness /'kɒnʃəsnɪs/ *n.* 意识

cerebellum /ˌserɪ'beləm/ *n.* 小脑

corticosteroid /ˌkɒtɪkəʊ'stɪərɒɪd/ *n.* 皮质类固醇

diuretic /ˌdaɪju'retɪk/ *n.* 利尿剂

anticonvulsant /ˌæntɪkən'vʌlsənt/ *n.* 抗惊厥的药物

seizure /'siːʒə/ *n.*（疾病）突然发作

Diabetes Mellitus

aneurysm /'ænjrɪzəm/ *n.* 动脉瘤

diabetes /ˌdaɪə'biːtiːz/ *n.* 糖尿病

metabolic /ˌmetə'bɒlɪk/ *adj.* 新陈代谢的

glucose /'gluːkəus/ *n.* 葡萄糖

insulin /'ɪnsjulɪn/ *n.* 胰岛素

microvascular /maɪkrəʊ'væskjulə/ *adj.* 微脉管的

atherosclerosis /ˌæθərəʊsklɪ'rəusɪs/ *n.* 动脉硬化症

coronary /'kɒrənəri/ *adj.* 冠状的

dehydration /ˌdiːhaɪ'dreɪʃ ən/ *n.* 脱水

hormone /'hɔː(r)məun/ *n.* 荷尔蒙，激素

vaginal /və'dʒaɪnəl/ *adj.* 阴道的

fluctuation /ˌflʌktʃu'eɪʃən/ *n.* 波动

onset /'ɒnset/ *n.* 发作

autoimmune /ˌɔːtəʊɪ'mjuːn/ *adj.* 自体免疫的

nephropathy /nə'frɒpəθɪ/ *n.* 肾病

neuropathy /njuə'rəpəθɪ/ *n.* 神经病

retinopathy /retɪ'nɒpəθɪ/ *n.* 视网膜病

fasting /'fɑːstɪŋ/ *adj.* 空腹的

cholesterol /kə'lestərɒl/ *n.* 胆固醇

Unit Five

Part 2　Listening and Speaking

Collecting Medical History

delicacy /'delɪkəsi/ *n.* 佳肴

Administering Medications

temptation /temp'teɪʃ ən/ *n.* 诱惑

deteriorate /dɪ'tɪərɪəreɪt/ *v.*（使）恶化

Part 3　Reading Comprehension

CT

opacify /əu'pæsɪfaɪ/ *vt.* 使……变得不透明

barium /'beəriəm/ *n.* 钡

dye /daɪ/ *n.* 碘剂

enema /'enɪmə/ *n.* 灌肠剂

gynecological /ˌgaɪnəkə'lɒdʒɪkəl/ *adj.* 妇产科医学的

intravenous /ˌɪntrə'viːnəs/ *adj.* 通过静脉的

contrast agent 造影剂

conspicuous /kən'spɪkjuəs/ *adj.* 显著的

Peptic Ulcer

sensation /sen'seɪʃ ən/ *n.* 感觉

impaired /ɪm'peəd/ *adj.* 受损的

glucophage /'gluːkəufeɪdʒ/ *n.* 盐酸二甲双胍

rotate /rəu'teɪt/ *vi.* 旋转

radiologist /ˌreɪdi'ɒlədʒɪst/ *n.* 放射医师

duodenum /ˌdjuːə'diːnəm/ *n.* 十二指肠

Helicobacter pylori 幽门螺旋杆菌

hydrochloric acid /ˌhaɪdrə'klɒrɪk 'æsɪd/ 氢氯酸，盐酸

enzyme /'enzaɪm/ *n.* 酶

pepsin /'pepsɪn/ *n.* 胃蛋白酶

mucous /'mjuːkəs/ *adj.* 黏液的

prostaglandin /ˌprɒstə'glændɪŋ/ *n.* 前列腺素

bacterium /bæk'tɪəriəm/ *n.* 细菌（复数为 bacteria）

prone /prəun/ *adj.* 倾向于

steroid /'stɪərɒɪd/ *n.* 类固醇

naproxen /nə'prɒksɪn/ *n.* 萘普生

ibuprofen /ˌaɪbju:'prəufen/ *n.* 布洛芬

antacid /ænt'æsɪd/ *n.* 抗酸剂

bloat /bləut/ *vi.* 膨胀

indicator /'ɪndɪkeɪtə/ *n.* 指示物

specimen /'spesɪmɪn/ *n.* 样本

organism /'ɔːgənɪzəm/ *n.* 生物体，有机体

antigen /'æntɪdʒən/ *n.* 抗原

Acute Kidney Failure

endoscopy /en'dɒskəpi/ *n.* 内窥镜检查法

esophagus /iː'sɒfəgəs/ *n.* 食道（oesophagus 的美式拼法）

penetrate /'penɪtreɪt/ *vt.* 穿透

perforation /pɜːfə'reɪʃ ən/ *n.* 穿孔

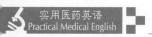
eliminate /ɪˈlɪmɪneɪt/ vt. 排除

disrupt /dɪsˈrʌpt/ vt. 使中断，破坏

reversible /rɪˈvɜːsəbl/ adj. 可逆的

overwhelming /ˌəʊvəˈwelmɪŋ/ adj. 无法抵抗的

retention /rɪˈtenʃən/ n. 潴留

pericarditis /ˌperɪkɑːˈdaɪtɪs/ n. 心包炎

inflammation /ˌɪnfləˈmeɪʃən/ n. 炎症

envelop /ɪnˈveləp/ vt. 包围

spine /spaɪn/ n. 脊柱，脊椎

aorta /eɪˈɔːtə/ n. 大动脉

oxygenate /ˈɒksɪdʒəneɪt/ vt. 氧化

nephron /ˈnefrɒn/ n. 肾单位，肾元

tuft /tʌft/ n. 一簇

capillary /kəˈpɪləri/ n. 毛细血管

glomerulus /gləʊˈmeərjuləs/ n. （肾）小球

tubule /ˈtjuːbjuːl/ n. 小管，细管

urea /juˈriːə/ n. 尿素

uric /ˈjuərɪk/ adj. 尿的

creatinine /kriːˈætɪniːn/ n. 肌氨酸酐

amino /əˈmiːnəu/ adj. 氨基的

Unit Six

Preoperative Instruction

preoperative /priːˈɒpərətɪv/ adj. 外科手术前的

appendectomy /ˌæpenˈdektəmi/ n. 阑尾切除术

Preoperative Nursing

anesthetic /ˌænəsˈθetɪk/ n. 麻醉剂

Part 3   Reading Comprehension

Overuse of Antibiotics

resistance /rɪˈzɪstəns/ n. 抵抗力

appendicitis /əˌpendɪˈsaɪtɪs/ n. 阑尾炎

appendix /əˈpendiks/ n. 阑尾

colon /ˈkəʊlən/ n. 结肠

Appendicitis

mutation /mjuːˈteɪʃən/ n. （生物细胞内的）突变

tuberculosis /tjuːˌbɜːkjʊˈləʊsɪs/ n. 结核病

germ /dʒɜːm/ n. 细菌，病菌

abdomen /ˈæbdəmən/ n. 腹部

characterize /ˈkærɪktəraɪz/ vt. 具有……的特征

blockage /ˈblɒkɪdʒ/ n. 阻塞

lumen /ˈluːmen/ n. 内腔

gangrene /ˈgæŋgriːn/ n. 坏疽

navel /ˈneɪvəl/ n. 肚脐

tenderness /ˈtendənɪs/ n. 柔和

palpate /ˈpælpeɪt/ vt. 触诊

lateral /ˈlætərəl/ adj. 横（向）的，侧面的

cecum /ˈsiːkəm/ n. 盲肠

flank /flæŋk/ n. 腰窝，肋腹

pelvis /ˈpelvɪs/ n. 骨盆

rectal /ˈrektəl/ adj. 直肠的

embryonic /ˌembrɪˈɒnɪk/ adj. 胚胎的

peritonitis /ˌperɪtəˈnaɪtɪs/ n. 腹膜炎

anesthesia /ˌænɪsˈθiːziə/ n. 麻醉（anasthesia 的美式拼法）

incision /ɪnˈsɪʒən/ n. （手术的）切痕，切口

laparoscopy /ˌlæpəˈrɒskəpɪ/ n. 腹腔镜检查

irrigate /ˈɪrɪgeɪt/ vt. 冲洗（伤口）

pus /pʌs/ n. 脓，脓汁

strenuous /ˈstrenjʊəs/ adj. 剧烈的

Constipation

constipation /ˌkɒnstɪˈpeɪʃən/ n. 便秘

bowel /ˈbaʊəl/ n. 肠

stool /stuːl/ n. 粪便

defecation /ˌdefəˈkeɪʃən/ n. 排便

contraction /kənˈtrækʃən/ n. （肌肉）挛缩

rectum /ˈrektəm/ n. 直肠

intake /ˈɪnteɪk/ n. 摄入量

pregnancy /ˈpregnənsi/ n. 怀孕

significant /sɪgˈnɪfɪkənt/ adj. 明显的

intestinal /ˌintesˈtaɪnl/ adj. 肠的

hypothyroidism /ˌhaɪpəʊˈθaɪrɔɪdɪzəm/ n. 甲状腺机能减退

electrolyte /ɪˈlektrəlaɪt/ n. 电解质

consume /kənˈsjuːm/ vt. 吃

linseed /ˈlɪnsiːd/ n. 亚麻子，亚麻仁

laxative /'læksətɪv/ *n.* 通便剂

stimulation /ˌstɪmju'leɪʃən/ *n.* 刺激

Unit Seven

Part 2 Listening and Speaking

Morning Shift Report

shift /ʃift/ *n.* 轮班

discharge /dɪs'tʃɑ:dʒ/ *vt.* 通知出院

admit /əd'mɪt/ *vt.* 接纳入院

Postoperative Nursing Discussion

acute /ə'kju:t/ *adj.* 急性的；严重的

chemotherapy /ˌki:məu'θerəpi/ *n.* 化学疗法

deceased /dɪ'si:st/ *adj.* 已故的

spleen /spli:n/ *n.* 脾脏

coma /'kəumə/ *n.* 昏迷

expire /ɪk'spaɪə/ *vi.* 死亡

complain /kəm'pleɪn/ *vi.* 述说有……病痛

intermittent /ˌɪntə'mɪtənt/ *adj.* 间歇的

Part 3 Reading Comprehension

Give Me a Break

fracture /'fræktʃə/ *n.* 骨折

comminute /'kɒmɪnju:t/ *vt.* 粉碎

compound /'kɒmpaund/ *n.* 混合体

react /rɪ'ækt/ *vi.* 反应

shock /ʃɒk/ *n.* 休克

X-ray /'eks reɪ/ *n.* X 光检查

metal plates 金属板

screw /skru:/ *n.* 螺钉

cast /kɑ:st/ *n.* 模型

bandage /'bændɪdʒ/ *n.* 绷带

heal /hi:l/ *vi.* 康复

splint /splɪnt/ *n.* 夹板

restrict /rɪs'trɪkt/ *vt.* 限制

calcium /'kælsiəm/ *n.* 钙

First Aid

provision /prə'vɪʒən/ *n.* 提供

lay /leɪ/ *adj.* 外行的

minimal /'mɪnɪməl/ *adj.* 极少的

collision /kə'lɪʒən/ *n.* 碰撞

overexertion /ˌəuvərɪg'zɜ:ʃən/ *n.* 努力过度

impair /ɪm'peə/ *vt.* 削弱，损害

choke /tʃəuk/ *vi.* 窒息

carotid /kə'rɒtɪd/ *n.* 颈动脉 *adj.* 颈动脉的

cardiopulmonary /ˌkɑ:dɪəu'pʌlmənərɪ/ *adj.* 心肺的

sequentially /sɪ'kwenʃəlɪ/ *adv.* 相继地，循序地

simultaneously /ˌsɪməl'teɪnɪəslɪ/ *adv.* 同时地

scrape /skreɪp/ *n.* 擦伤

rinse /rɪns/ *vt.* 冲洗

gauze /gɔ:z/ *n.* 纱布

Bone Fracture

partial /'pɑ:ʃəl/ *adj.* 局部的

crack /kræk/ *n.* 裂缝

transverse /trænz'vɜ:s/ *adj.* 横向的

oblique /ə'bli:k/ *adj.* 倾斜的

spiral /'spaɪərəl/ *adj.* 螺旋形的

multiple /'mʌltɪpl/ *adj.* 多重的

bruising /'bru:zɪŋ/ *n.* 瘀青

paralyze /'pærəlaɪz/ *vt.* 使瘫痪，使麻痹

tomography /tə'mɒgrəfi/ *n.* X 线断层摄影术

magnetic /mæg'netɪk/ *adj.* 有磁性的

resonance /'rezənəns/ *n.* 共振

immobilization /ɪˌməubəlaɪ'zeɪʃən/ *n.* 固定

surgery /'sɜ:dʒəri/ *n.* 外科手术

manipulate /mə'nɪpjuleɪt/ *vt.* (熟练地) 操作

alignment /ə'laɪnmənt/ *n.* 平行的排列

permanent /'pɜ:mənənt/ *adj.* 永久的

Unit Eight

Part 2 Listening and Speaking

Health Instruction

acquired /ə'kwaɪəd/ *adj.* 获得的，后天的

deficiency /dɪ'fɪʃənsɪ/ *n.* 不足

immunodeficiency /ˌɪmju:nəudɪ'fɪʃənsɪ/ *n.* 免疫缺陷

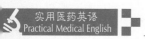

swollen /ˈswəʊlən/ *adj.* 肿胀的

lymph /lɪmf/ *n.* 淋巴

node /nəʊd/ *n.* 节点

Part 3　Reading Comprehension

Florence Nightingale

commemorate /kəˈmeməreɪt/ *vt.* 纪念

merciful /ˈmɜːsɪfəl/ *adj.* 慈悲的

sympathetic /ˌsɪmpəˈθetɪk/ *adj.* 有同情心的

sanitary /ˈsænɪtərɪ/ *adj.* 卫生的

Leukemia

theoretical /ˌθɪəˈretɪkəl/ *adj.* 理论的

excessive /ɪkˈsesɪv/ *adj.* 过度的

strain /streɪn/ *n.* 焦虑

respectable /rɪˈspektəbl/ *adj.* 受人尊敬的

funeral /ˈfjuːnərəl/ *n.* 葬礼

observe /əbˈzɜːv/ *vt.* 遵守

workshop /ˈwɜːkʃɒp/ *n.* 研讨会，工作坊

leukemia /luːˈkiːmɪə/ *n.* 白血病

malignant /məˈlɪgnənt/ *adj.* 恶性的

hematopoietic /hemətəʊpɒɪˈiːtɪk/ *adj.* 造血的

marrow /ˈmærəʊ/ *n.* 骨髓

lymphocytic /ˌlɪmfəˈsaɪtɪk/ *adj.* 淋巴细胞的

myelogenous /ˌmaɪəˈlɒdʒənəs/ *adj.* 骨髓性的

radiation /ˌreɪdɪˈeɪʃən/ *n.* 放射物

nuclein /ˈnjuːklɪɪn/ *n.* 核素

benzene /ˈbenziːn/ *n.* 苯

carcinogen /kɑːˈsɪnədʒən/ *n.* 致癌物

circulatory /sɜːkjʊˈleɪtərɪ/ *adj.* 血液循环的

dope /dəʊp/ *n.* 涂料

lacquer /ˈlækə/ *n.* 漆

solvent /ˈsɒlvənt/ *n.* 溶剂

immature /ˌɪməˈtʃʊə/ *adj.* 不成熟的

clot /klɒt/ *vi.* 凝结

anemia /əˈniːmɪə/ *n.* 贫血

dyspnea /dɪsˈpniːə/ *n.* 呼吸困难

neurological /ˌnjʊərəˈlɒdʒɪkəl/ *adj.* 神经学的

diarrhea /ˌdaɪəˈrɪə/ *n.* 腹泻

AIDS

attribute /əˈtrɪbjuːt/ *vt.* 把……归因于

transplantation /ˌtrænsplɑːnˈteɪʃn/ *n.* 移植

superficial /suːpəˈfɪʃəl/ *adj.* 表皮的

lymphadenopathy /ˈlɪmˌfædəˈnɒpəθɪ/ *n.* 淋巴结病

anorexia /ˌænəˈreksɪə/ *n.* 厌食

hemiplegia /ˌhemɪˈpliːdʒɪə/ *n.* 偏瘫

dementia /dɪˈmenʃə/ *n.* 痴呆

herpes /ˈhɜːpiːz/ *n.* 疱疹

zoster /ˈzɒstə/ *n.* 带，带状疹子

ulceration /ˌʌlsəˈreɪʃən/ *n.* 溃疡

macula /ˈmækjʊlə/ *n.* 斑疹

immunoassay /ˌɪmjʊnəʊˈæseɪ/ *n.* 免疫测定

condom /ˈkɒndəm/ *n.* 避孕套

prenatal /ˌpriːˈneɪtl/ *adj.* 产前的

Unit Nine

Part 2　Listening and Speaking

Discharge

armpit /ˈɑːmˌpɪt/ *n.* 腋窝

Health Education

aerobic /ˌeəˈrəʊbɪk/ *adj.* 有氧的

Part 3　Reading Comprehension

Childhood Obesity

obesity /əʊˈbiːsətɪ/ *n.* 肥胖

adolescent /ˌædəʊˈlesənt/ *n.* 青少年

triple /ˈtrɪpl/ *vi.* 增至三倍

decade /ˈdekeɪd/ *n.* 十年

ignore /ɪgˈnɔː/ *vt.* 忽视

crucial /ˈkruːʃəl/ *adj.* 极重要的

highlight /ˈhaɪlaɪt/ *vt.* 强调

stipulate /ˈstɪpjəleɪt/ *vt.* 要求

Obesity

forum /ˈfɔːrəm/ *n.* 论坛

premise /ˈpremɪs/ *n.* 前提

neglect /nɪˈglekt/ *n.* 疏忽

malnutrition /ˌmælnjuˈtrɪʃ ən/ *n.* 营养不良

overweight /ˌəʊvəˈweɪt/ *n.* 超重

calorie /ˈkælərɪ/ *n.* 卡路里

metric /ˈmetrɪk/ *n.* 度量标准

obese /əʊˈbiːs/ *adj.* 肥胖的

morbidly /ˈmɔːbɪdlɪ/ *adv.* 病态地

appetite /ˈæpɪtaɪt/ *n.* 食欲

osteoarthritis /ˌɒstɪəʊɑːˈθraitis/ *n.* 骨关节炎

degeneration /dɪˌdʒenəˈreɪʃ ən/ *n.* 恶化

cartilage /ˈkɑːtilidʒ/ *n.* 软骨

gallbladder /ˈgɔːlˌblædə/ *n.* 胆囊

apnea /ˈæpniə/ *n.* 无呼吸，呼吸暂停

endometrial /endʌˈmetriəl/ *adj.* 子宫内膜的

perceive /pəˈsiːv/ *vt.* 察觉

mobilize /ˈməʊbɪlaɪz/ *vt.* 调动

Stress

hypothalamus /ˌhaɪpəˈθæləməs/ *n.* 下丘脑

adrenal /əˈdriːnl/ *adj.* 肾上腺的

cortisol /ˈkɔːtisɒl/ *n.* 皮质醇

overreact /ˌəʊvərɪˈækt/ *vi.* 反应过度

contradict /ˌkɒntrəˈdɪkt/ *vt.* 否认……的真实性

distract /dɪˈstrækt/ *vt.* 使分心

Unit Ten

Part 2   Listening and Speaking

Administration of Medication

oral /ˈɔːrəl/ *adj.* 口的，口腔的

tablet /ˈtæblɪt/ *n.* 药片

external /ɪkˈstɜːnl/ *adj.* 外用的

ointment /ˈɔɪntmənt/ *n.* 药膏

adverse /ˈædvɜːs/ *adj.* 不利的

Part 3   Reading Comprehension

Attention to Mental Health

observance /əbˈzɜːvəns/ *n.*（对风俗或仪式的）遵守

schizophrenia /ˌskɪtsəʊˈfriːnɪə/ *n.* 精神分裂症

alcohol /ˈælkəhɒl/ *n.* 酒精

abuse /əˈbjuːs/ *n.* 滥用

affect /əˈfekt/ *vt.* 影响

enormous /ɪˈnɔːməs/ *adj.* 巨大的

access /ˈækses/ *n.* 通道

stigma /ˈstɪgmə/ *n.* 耻辱

percentage /pəˈsentɪdʒ/ *n.* 百分比

communicable /kəˈmjuːnɪkəbl/ *adj.* 可传染的

capacity /kəˈpæsɪtɪ/ *n.* 能力

availability /əˌveɪləˈbɪlɪtɪ/ *n.* 有效性

psychosocial /ˌsaɪkəʊˈsəʊʃəl/ *adj.* 社会心理的

vulnerable /ˈvʌlnərəbəl/ *adj.* 易受伤害的

exclude /ɪksˈkluːd/ *vt.* 排斥

Coronary Heart Disease

approximately /əˈprɒksɪˈmətlɪ/ *adv.* 大约

vein /veɪn/ *n.* 静脉

circulation /ˌsɜːkjuˈleɪʃ ən/ *n.* 循环

vessel /ˈvesl/ *n.* 脉管

artery /ˈɑːtərɪ/ *n.* 动脉

partially /ˈpɑːʃəlɪ/ *adv.* 部分地

angina /ænˈdʒaɪnə/ *n.* 心绞痛

myocardial /ˌmaɪəʊˈkɑːdɪəl/ *adj.* 心肌的

infarction /ɪnˈfɑːkʃ ən/ *n.* 梗塞（梗死）形成

palpitation /pælpɪˈteɪʃ ən/ *n.* 心悸

unduly /ʌnˈdjuːlɪ/ *adv.* 过度地

cholesterol /kəˈlestərəʊl/ *n.* 胆固醇

thrombosis /θrɒmˈbəʊsɪs/ *n.* 血栓症

atheroma /æθəˈrəʊmə/ *n.* 动脉粥样化

Hypertension

bypass /ˈbaɪpɑːs/ *n.* 旁通管

transplant /trænsˈplɑːnt/ *n.* 移植

consumption /kənˈsʌmpʃ ən/ *n.* 消费

hypertension /ˌhaɪpəˈtenʃ ən/ *n.* 高血压

afflict /əˈflɪkt/ *vt.* 折磨

asymptomatic /ˌeɪsɪmptəˈmætɪk/ *adj.* 无症状的

stroke /strəʊk/ *n.* 中风

dysfunction /dɪsˈfʌŋkʃ ən/ *n.* 功能紊乱

systolic /ˌsɪsˈtɒlɪk/ *adj.* 心脏收缩的

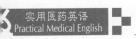

diastolic /ˌdaɪəˈstɒlɪk/ *adj.* 心脏舒张的

value /ˈvæljuː/ *n.* (数)值

primary /ˈpraɪmərɪ/ *adj.* 原发性的

identifiable /aɪˈdentɪfaɪəbl/ *adj.* 可以确认的

secondary /ˈsekəndərɪ/ *adj.* 继发性的

category /ˈkætɪgərɪ/ *n.* 种类

potassium /pəˈtæsjəm/ *n.* 钾

antihypertensive /ˌæntɪˌhaɪpəˈtensɪv/ *adj.* 抗高血
压的

cardiac /ˈkɑːdɪæk/ *adj.* 心脏的

vasodilator /ˌvæsəʊdaɪˈleɪtə/ *adj.* 血管扩张的

systemic /sɪsˈtemɪk/ *adj.* 全身的

vascular /ˈvæskjulə/ *adj.* 血管的

unprocessed /ˌʌnˈprəʊsest/ *adj.* 未被加工的

7. Vocabulary

A

B

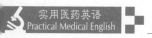

D

decade /'dekeɪd/ *n.* 十年 (125)

deceased /dɪ'siːst/ *adj.* 已故的 (94)

decongestant /ˌdiːkən'dʒestənt/ *n.* 减充血剂 (25)

defecation /ˌdefə'keɪʃən/ *n.* 排便 (83)

deficiency /dɪ'fɪʃənsi/ *n.* 不足 (108)

definition /ˌdefɪ'nɪʃən/ *n.* 定义 (8)

degeneration /dɪˌdʒenə'reɪʃən/ *n.* 恶化 (129)

dehydration /ˌdiːhaɪ'dreɪʃən/ *n.* 脱水 (55)

delicacy /'delɪkəsi/ *n.* 佳肴 (64)

dementia /dɪ'menʃə/ *n.* 痴呆 (115)

dentist /'dentɪst/ *n.* 牙科医生 (19)

deteriorate /dɪ'tɪəriəreɪt/ *v.*(使）恶化 (65)

detrimental /ˌdetrɪ'mentl/ *adj.* 有害的 (40)

diabetes /ˌdaɪə'biːtiːz/ *n.* 糖尿病 (55)

diagnosis /ˌdaɪəg'nəʊsɪs/ *n.* 诊断 (52)

diagnostic /ˌdaɪəg'nɒstɪk/ *adj.* 诊断的 (51)

diaphragm /'daɪəfræm/ *n.* 横膈膜 (10)

diarrhea /ˌdaɪə'rɪə/ *n.* 腹泻 (113)

diastolic /ˌdaɪə'stɒlɪk/ *adj.* 心脏舒张的 (147)

differentiation /ˌdɪfəˌrenʃɪ'eɪʃən/ *n.* 分化 (9)

digestion /daɪ'dʒestʃən/ *n.* 消化 (9)

digestive /daɪ'dʒestɪv/ *adj.* 消化的 (8)

dioxide /daɪ'ɒksaɪd/ *n.* 二氧化物 (6)

discharge /dɪs'tʃɑːdʒ/ *vt.* 通知出院 (93)

disrupt /dɪs'rʌpt/ *vt.* 使中断，破坏 (69)

disruption /dɪs'rʌpʃən/ *n.* 破坏 (9)

distinctive /dɪs'tɪŋktɪv/ *adj.* 有特色的 (10)

distract /dɪ'strækt/ *vt.* 使分心 (131)

distress /dɪs'tres/ *n.* 窘迫 (42)

diuretic /ˌdaɪjʊ'retɪk/ *n.* 利尿剂 (54)

domesticate /də'mestɪkeɪt/ *vt.* 驯养（动物） (41)

dope /dəʊp/ *n.* 涂料 (113)

drainage /'dreɪnɪdʒ/ *n.* 引流 (24)

duodenum /ˌdjuːə'diːnəm/ *n.* 十二指肠 (67)

dye /daɪ/ *n.* 碘剂 (66)

dysfunction /dɪs'fʌŋkʃən/ *n.* 功能紊乱 (147)

dyspnea /dɪs'pniːə/ *n.* 呼吸困难 (113)

E

edema /ɪ'diːmə/ *n.* 浮肿，水肿 (27)

effusion /ɪ'fjuːʒən/ *n.* 流出物 (27)

electrolyte /ɪ'lektrəlaɪt/ *n.* 电解质 (84)

eliminate /ɪ'lɪmɪneɪt/ *vt.* 排除 (69)

embryonic /ˌembrɪ'ɒnɪk/ *adj.* 胚胎的 (82)

emphysema /ˌemfɪ'siːmə/ *n.* 肺气肿 (24)

endocrine /'endəʊkrɪn/ *n.* 内分泌 (8)

endometrial /endʌ'metriəl/ *adj.* 子宫内膜的 (129)

endoscopy /en'dɒskəpi/ *n.* 内窥镜检查法 (69)

enema /'enɪmə/ *n.* 灌肠剂 (66)

enormous /ɪ'nɔːməs/ *adj.* 巨大的 (143)

envelop /ɪn'veləp/ *vt.* 包围 (70)

enzyme /'enzaɪm/ *n.* 酶 (67)

epithelial /ˌepɪ'θiːliəl/ *adj.* 上皮的 (8)

esophagus /iː'sɒfəgəs/ *n.* 食道（oesophagus 的美式拼法） (69)

ester /'estə/ *n.* 酯 (22)

excessive /ɪk'sesɪv/ *adj.* 过度的 (111)

exclude /ɪks'kluːd/ *vt.* 排斥 (144)

excretion /ɪk'skriːʃən/ *n.* 排泄 (11)

expire /ɪk'spaɪə/ *vi.* 死亡 (94)

external /ɪk'stɜːnl/ *adj.* 外用的 (141)

F

fasting /'fɑːstɪŋ/ *adj.* 空腹的 (57)

fatigue /fə'tiːg/ *n.* 疲劳 (26)

feces /'fiːsiːz/ *n.* 粪便，排泄物 (41)

feed /fiːd/ *n.* 饲料 (42)

fertilize /'fɜːtɪlaɪz/ *vt.* 使受精 (8)

flank /flæŋk/ *n.* 腰窝，肋腹 (82)

fluctuation /ˌflʌktʃu'eɪʃən/ *n.* 波动 (56)

fluid /'fluːɪd/ *n.* 流体 (22)

forum /'fɔːrəm/ *n.* 论坛 (127)

fracture /'fræktʃə/ *n.* 骨折 (95)

fundamental /ˌfʌndə'mentl/ *n.* 基本原则 (4)

funeral /'fjuːnərəl/ *n.* 葬礼 (111)

fungi /'fʌŋdʒaɪ/ *n.*(fungus 的复数）真菌 (26)

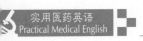

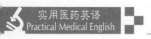

react /rɪˈækt/ *vi.* 反应 (95)

rectal /ˈrektəl/ *adj.* 直肠的 (82)

rectum /ˈrektəm/ *n.* 直肠 (83)

recur /rɪˈkɜː/ *vi.* 复发 (24)

remedy /ˈremɪdi/ *n.* 疗法 (52)

replacement /rɪˈpleɪsmənt/ *n.* 代替 (10)

reproductive /ˌriːprəˈdʌktɪv/ *adj.* 生殖的 (8)

resistance /rɪˈzɪstəns/ *n.* 抵抗力 (79)

resistant /rɪˈzɪstənt/ *adj.* 有耐药性的 (42)

resonance /ˈrezənəns/ *n.* 共振 (100)

respectable /rɪˈspektəbl/ *adj.* 受人尊敬的 (111)

respiration /ˌrespəˈreɪʃən/ *n.* 呼吸 (9)

respiratory /rɪˈspɪrətəri/ *adj.* 呼吸的 (8)

restrict /rɪsˈtrɪkt/ *vt.* 限制 (96)

retention /rɪˈtenʃən/ *n.* 潴留 (70)

retinopathy /retɪˈnɒpəθɪ/ *n.* 视网膜病 (57)

reversible /rɪˈvɜːsəbl/ *adj.* 可逆的 (69)

ribavirin /raɪbəˈvaɪərɪn/ *n.* 病毒唑（抗病毒药） (40)

rinse /rɪns/ *vt.* 冲洗 (98)

rotate /rəʊˈteɪt/ *vi.* 旋转 (67)

rupture /ˈrʌptʃə/ *n.* 破裂 (53)

S

saliva /səˈlaɪvə/ *n.* 唾液 (41)

sanitary /ˈsɜnɪtəri/ *adj.* 卫生的 (110)

schizophrenia /ˌskɪtsəʊˈfriːnɪə/ *n.* 精神分裂症 (143)

scrape /skreɪp/ *n.* 擦伤 (98)

screw /skruː/ *n.* 螺钉 (96)

secondary /ˈsekəndərɪ/ *adj.* 继发性的 (148)

secretion /siˈkriːʃən/ *n.* 分泌物 (41)

seizure /ˈsiːʒə/ *n.* （疾病）突然发作 (54)

sensation /senˈseɪʃən/ *n.* 感觉 (67)

sensitivity /ˌsensɪˈtɪvɪti/ *n.* 灵敏性 (27)

sequentially /sɪˈkwenʃəlɪ/ *adv.* 相继地，循序地 (98)

shift /ʃift/ *n.* 轮班 (93)

shock /ʃɒk/ *n.* 休克 (96)

significant /sɪgˈnɪfɪkənt/ *adj.* 明显的 (84)

simultaneously /ˌsɪməlˈteɪnɪəslɪ/ *adv.* 同时地 (98)

sinus /ˈsaɪnəs/ *n.* 窦 (24)

skeletal /ˈskelɪtl/ *adj.* 骨骼的 (8)

soluble /ˈsɒljʊbl/ *adj.* 可溶的 (6)

solvent /ˈsɒlvənt/ *n.* 溶剂 (113)

sophomore /ˈsɒfəmɔː/ *n.* 大学二年级学生 (4)

specimen /ˈspesɪmɪn/ *n.* 样本 (68)

spine /spaɪn/ *n.* 脊柱，脊椎 (70)

spiral /ˈspaɪərəl/ *adj.* 螺旋形的 (99)

spleen /spliːn/ *n.* 脾脏 (94)

splint /splɪnt/ *n.* 夹板 (96)

spray /spreɪ/ *n.* 喷雾 (25)

starch /staːtʃ/ *n.* 淀粉 (22)

sterilization /sterɪlaɪˈzeɪʃən/ *n.* 杀菌 (4)

steroid /ˈstɪərɒɪd/ *n.* 类固醇 (68)

stigma /ˈstɪgmə/ *n.* 耻辱 (143)

stimulation /ˌstɪmjʊˈleɪʃən/ *n.* 刺激 (85)

stimulus /ˈstɪmjʊləs/ *n.* 刺激 (10)

stipulate /ˈstɪpjəleɪt/ *vt.* 要求 (126)

stool /stuːl/ *n.* 粪便 (83)

strain /streɪn/ *n.* 焦虑 (111)

strenuous /ˈstrenjʊəs/ *adj.* 剧烈的 (82)

stroke /strəʊk/ *n.* 中风 (147)

subsequently /ˈsʌbsɪkwəntli/ *adv.* 后来 (26)

superficial /suːpəˈfɪʃəl/ *adj.* 表皮的 (115)

supplemental /ˌsʌpliˈmentl/ *adj.* 补足的 (40)

surgeon /ˈsɜːdʒən/ *n.* 外科医生 (19)

surgery /ˈsɜːdʒəri/ *n.* 外科手术 (100)

surgical /ˈsɜːdʒɪkəl/ *adj.* 外科的 (4)

survival /səˈvaɪvəl/ *n.* 生存 (8)

susceptible /səˈseptəbl/ *adj.* 易受影响的 (41)

swelling /ˈswelɪŋ/ *n.* 肿胀 (54)

swollen /ˈswəʊlən/ *adj.* 肿胀的 (108)

sympathetic /ˌsɪmpəˈθetɪk/ *adj.* 有同情心的 (110)

syndrome /ˈsɪndrəʊm/ *n.* 症状 (39)

systemic /sɪsˈtemɪk/ *adj.* 全身的 (149)

systolic /ˌsɪsˈtɒlɪk/ *adj.* 心脏收缩的 (147)

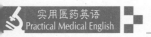